A
Short History
of
Clinical Midwifery

The Development of Ideas in the
Professional Management of Childbirth

Philip Rhodes

Emeritus Professor
MA, MB, BChir(Cantab.), FRCS(Eng.), FRCOG,
FRACMA, FFOM(RCP), FRSA

Books for Midwives Press
Books for Midwives Press is a joint publishing collaboration
between The Royal College of Midwives and
Haigh & Hochland Publications Ltd

Published by Books for Midwives Press, 174a Ashley Road, Hale, Cheshire, WA15 9SF, England

First edition

ISBN 1-898507-22-8

British Library Cataloguing in Publication Data
A catalogue record for this book is available from the British Library

Printed in Great Britain by Cromwell Press Ltd

Contents

List of Illustrations

Chapter Three

Figure 3.1: *Fetus in Utero* by Soranus from *An Outline History of Medicine,* by Philip Rhodes, Butterworths, 1985.

Chapter Four

Figure 4.1: An Obstetrical Chair from *Devils, Drugs and Doctors,* by Howard W. Haggard. By permission of Wm. Heinemann (Medical Books) Ltd.

Figure 4.2: A Baptismal Syringe from *Deveils, Drugs and Doctors,* by Howard W. Haggard. By permission of Wm. Heinemann (Medical Books) Ltd.

Figure 4.3: Frontispiece of *Der Swangeren Frauen und Hebammen Rosengarten'* from *Eternal Eve* by Harvey Graham. By permission of Wm. Heinemann (Medical Books) Ltd, 1950.

Figure 4.4: Frontispiece of *De Conceptu et Generatione Hominis'*. Reproduced by courtesy of the Library of the Royal College of Obstetricians and Gynaecologists.

Figure 4.5: *Fetus in utero* by Leonardo da Vinci. From *An Outline History of Medicine* by Philip Rhodes, Butterworths, 1985.

Figure 4.6: Frontispiece from *The Byrth of Mankind.* Courtesy of the Library of the Royal College of Obstetricians and Gynaecologists.

Figure 4.7: Portrait of Ambroise Paré from *An Outline History of Medicine* by Philip Rhodes, Butterworths, 1985.

Chapter Five

Figure 5.1: Portrait of William Harvey from *An Outline History of Medicine* by Philip Rhodes, Butterworths, 1985.

Figure 5.2: Portrait of Louise Bourgeois. Courtesy of the Library of the Royal College of Obstetricians and Gynaecologists.

Figure 5.3: Portrait of Justine Siegemundin. Courtesy of the Library of the Royal College of Obstetricians and Gynaecologists.

Figure 5.4: First and title pages from *Observations in Midwifery* by Percivall Willughby, 1596–1685.

Figure 5.5: Hooks or crotchets from *La Commare o Riccoglitrice.* Courtesy of the Library of the Royal College of Obstetricians and Gynaecologists.

Figure 5.6: Lever. Courtesy of the Library of the Royal College of Obstetricians and Gynaecologists.

Figure 5.7: Speculum matricis from *De Conceptu et Generatione Hominis.* Courtesy of the Library of the Royal College of Obstetricians and Gynaecologists.

Chapter Six

Figure 6.1: Chapman's Forceps from his *Treatise on Midwifery,* John Brindley, London, 1735.

Chapter Seven

Chapter Eight

Chapter Nine

Acknowledgements

There are many to whom I owe a debt in the writing of this book. My wife has become used to me being closeted in my study in front of the word processor, and patiently accepts this. At least it keeps me from being under her feet in my retirement.

Obtaining pictures for reproduction in a book is always a chore of the most unforgiving, time-consuming kind. In this troublesome task I have been enormously helped by the willing, cheerful and ever-helpful Patricia Want, Librarian of the Royal College of Obstetricians and Gynaecologists. I cannot thank her enough.

Above all I am grateful to previous authors on midwifery and obstetric themes and history.

Preface

There have been no general histories of clinical midwifery for about 40 years. Among the best were Harvey Graham's *Eternal Eve* (1950) and *Historical Review of British Obstetrics and Gynaecology1800–1950* (1954). This was to supplement *The History of British Midwifery: from 1650 to 1800* (1927) by Herbert R. Spencer. There have been many others on specialized parts of the history of midwifery, often lavishly produced in America. More recently medical history has been taken over by historians, often with sociological and other biases, rather than clinical ones. These historians' works often show ignorance and inadequate consideration and understanding of the clinical work done by midwives and obstetricians.

So there have not been any brief reviews of the general historical progress of clinical midwifery and its offspring, obstetrics, for many years, which could be of interest to ordinary men and women, as well as their various helpers in matters of childbearing. Hopefully this book will fill a gap in midwifery and general education, and lead to an awakened interest in the subject matter, which has been neglected for some time.

Over the centuries millions of women have suffered and died in childbirth and during childbearing. In the western world, with which this book is mainly concerned, it is safer to have a baby now – in terms of maternal mortality and morbidity – than it has ever been. Babies, too, have a much better prognosis than heretofore.

Those happier outcomes have come about through better hygiene, nutrition and education of mothers as well as the work of many pioneers who have struggled to overcome the clinical problems of their times. In that struggle there have been both successes and failures. Progress in science and technology is seldom seen in a straight line, but is more like a meandering river. That is how it has been in midwifery, yet there really has been progress. This book is a sketch of that progress in the conquest of difficult labour, pain, haemorrhage and infection, as well as eclampsia, and many other things. It is a history of the ideas that have developed about all of them. Much has been done. Much remains to do. But it may be of interest to know how we have come to the present situation in the theory and practice of the clinical management of childbirth in all its phases.

CHAPTER ONE

The Beginnings

The origins of civilisation lie in Mesopotamia, in the land between the Tigris and the Euphrates in modern Iraq and Turkey. There were nomadic tribes and a few settlements. It is difficult to guess at their understanding of childbirth, but they must have known about reproduction in their animals and learned something from that. In butchering they must sometimes have seen a fetus and placenta in the womb, and have associated that with pregnancy in the women of their more nomadic tribes. However, because of the turmoil of labour they probably subscribed to the ancient view that the fetus fought its way out of the womb by its own efforts. It was these that were thought to cause the mother so much distress. An outstanding feature of childbirth is the way in which the pain almost ceases as soon as the child is born, so it was a reasonable assumption then that the fetus was the cause of the pain.

Men were not involved with any aspects of reproduction except fertilisation. It has been suggested that the primitive peoples did not associate intercourse with pregnancy, but this seems unlikely. It was obviously known to be so associated in animals, and there must have been awareness of the early symptoms of amenorrhoea, morning sickness, and breast changes shortly after intercourse.

Women had to look after their own. Some would have come to some expertise in the management of labour and the caring for the newborn. But of course there could be no understanding of bleeding in pregnancy nor of fits. Pain had to be borne with no relief and obstructed labour and bleeding after birth were terrors about which nothing could be done. One can only surmise that maternal, fetal and neonatal mortalities were considerably higher than those of today. It is a myth that primitive childbirth is simple and straightforward. Evidence from all over the present third world shows that this is not so. Many women in underdeveloped countries suffer untold horrors and frequently die in pregnancy, in labour and in the puerperium. They are certainly not as well protected as women of the western world from their childbearing perils.

Yet there is no doubt that statistically, through the ages, childbirth has been all too successful. The world population goes on rising and rising, and by some that is deemed to be the beginnings of catastrophe. But midwifery's main concern is with individual women and how they may best be cared for. Its driving force is to make as sure as possible that both mother and baby healthily survive what can be a potentially dangerous experience or both of them.

Hellenic times

The centres of culture and civilisation moved up the Tigris and Euphrates and from Egypt via Crete to Ionia on the western shore of the Aegean Sea. There Greek (Hellenic) culture began, and over the centuries it developed further in the city states of mainland

Greece. The organization of society was such that there was a leisured class which devoted itself to philosophy, science and mathematics among many other intellectual pursuits. These though were the preserves of men, and women's interests were subsidiary. There was therefore little concern with affairs of childbirth, except there could be supplications to the goddess Hera, the wife of Zeus, who was the deity for marriage and childbirth. Later there could be similar supplications to Artemis, or Diana in the Roman pantheon, and to Eileithyia, known as the 'girdle-loosener', who could be invoked to alleviate the pains of childbirth.

Medicine was a matter of folklore and was practised, if at all, by members of the slave class. Yet a few men of the educated classes did begin to study the subject rather as an adjunct to philosophy and science. Among them was the Father of Medicine, Hippocrates. He was born about 460 BC and lived for about 60 years. He practised mainly on the island of Cos, lying off the coast of modern Turkey, which was Ionia. He was known to Plato and was a contemporary of Socrates. He founded a school on Cos to which people came from far and wide to learn his theory and practice.

Although he was an historical person the Hippocratic tradition lasted for several hundred years, so he is not the sole author of the 60 or so treatises in the Hippocratic Collection, which includes *The Seed* and *The Nature of the Child*. These attempt to grapple with the problems of conception and development in the womb. Because exact knowledge of anatomy and physiology were lacking in comparison with today there were few relevant insights to the present.

The Seed considered that the 'sperm' came from all the fluid in the body, and was the most potent of them all. Ejaculation of semen was believed to cause weakness, a belief still persisting in some quarters today, but entirely without foundation. There follows a hotchpotch of ideas about warmth and foam and fluid diffusing from the brain, through the spinal marrow, on to the kidneys and then to the testes. It was even thought that a cut behind the ear would result in sterility.

Women were deemed to have less pleasure in sexual intercourse than men. They produced a discharge which was thought to be female semen. These male and female seminal fluids were mixed together in the womb and there developed into a baby. 'Strong' semen from either sex resulted in the formation of a male and 'weak' semen in a female. Small babies at birth resulted from escape of discharge from the womb which was thought to be nourishment of which the baby is deprived. There are many other speculative comments, but they should not be derided for they were a sincere attempt to understand difficult phenomena in the light of knowledge of the times.

The Nature of the Child attempted explanations of the development of the baby on the basis of breath (air) and heat and cold. These notions of development came from the four elements of earth, air, fire and water, the four *humours* (liquids) of which the body is made – blood, phlegm, white bile and black bile – and the four *qualities* of hot, cold, dry and moist. This elaborate theory held medicine in thrall for several hundred years. Virtually everything medical had to be forced into conformation with this erroneous theoretical mould.

However, the author of *The Nature* had seen an aborted embryo. He thought it looked like a hen's egg from which the shell had been removed. From his observation he speculated that nourishment reaches the baby by a flux of blood every day, and he related this to menstruation, which was caused by changes in temperature every month. When the woman was full of blood she could not conceive but when emptied by menstruation she could. This led to the belief that the best time for conception was just after menstruation, yet another belief wrongly perpetuated from these early times.

Labour, according to this author, was caused by the blood becoming agitated and warm. The baby was stirred up and then by its vigorous movements broke the membranes and proceeded to force its way out of the womb by its own efforts. Partly this belief was based on observations of the chick which pecks its way out of the egg. It exemplifies an analogical argument which is now manifestly false.

Further observations and speculations are made on the breasts. It was thought that milk nourished the baby during pregnancy. It was known that if the breasts suddenly slackened then a miscarriage was likely to be imminent. There is a section which reads: 'A male foetus inclines to the right, a female to the left.' There are people who still seem to believe this. Without detailing all the various aphorisms perhaps enough has been said to show that there were glimpses of the truth about childbirth amidst a welter of totally inaccurate speculation. But science had not then advanced to the stage of attempting to ground speculation in fact.

In *Epidemics* there are several descriptions of women who suffered from puerperal fever. As clinical case histories they are remarkably accurate. Nearly all of the women died.

Strangely, almost nothing was written about labour. This is probably because the literate gentlemen who wrote the Hippocratic canon did not supervise labour which was deemed to be a matter for other women and perhaps slaves. Vaginal examinations seem to have been carried out rarely and abdominal examination almost not at all. One oddity that has persisted is that it was thought valuable to make the woman sneeze in order to expel the placenta.

Despite the many erroneous speculations and the relative paucity of direct clinical observation these early pioneer authors deserve their meed of praise. They began to progress from complete ignorance and ground some of their speculations in clinical observations. This was a great advance for medicine as a whole, though perhaps not for midwifery. Moreover the speculations and observations were written down so that others could learn from them and build on them. It was the start of refining folklore and custom which was all that had previously been present. It began too to define a 'professional' class with special interests in medicine as well as philosophy.

A full treatment of the Hippocratic Collection is given in *Hippocratic Writings*, edited by Lloyd, G.E.R., translated by Chadwick J. and Mann, W.N., and published by Penguin Books, London, 1978.

CHAPTER TWO

The Bible

The Bible has been responsible for many of the attitudes to women in christian countries of the western world. There is the famous curse of Eve from Genesis, 'In sorrow shalt thou bring forth'. It was she who was thought to be entirely responsible for the Fall of Man, by getting Adam to eat the fruit of the Tree of Knowledge. It is an unmerited curse, unworthy of modern concepts of God, and it has done untold harm to the cause of women throughout the ages.

A more modern translation from *The New International Version of the Holy Bible* (1978) is,

> 'I will greatly increase your pains in childbearing; with pain will you give birth to children; Your desire will be for your husband, and he will rule over you.'

This is slightly softer than the original version, and is an attempt to explain the pain of labour and the subservience of women to men in theological terms. It seeks too to justify as God-given the cultural attitudes of the relationships between husbands and wives at the time the text was written.

Sarai, the wife of Abraham, was infertile, so her Egyptian handmaiden was induced to sleep with Abraham, and she bore Ishmael. This is an interesting example of surrogacy, for the children of servants and slaves were accepted as children of the head of the household. However, despite her age, Sarah, as she was later called, did bear a son called Isaac. The family was then living in Canaan. In order to avoid Isaac marrying a girl from there a messenger was dispatched to Abraham's tribe, where Rebekah was found as she drew water from the well at Nahor. It was she who bore twins, Esau and Jacob, to Isaac. Rebekah favoured Jacob over Esau and deceived her husband into giving the birthright to Jacob, when the older twin was Esau.

Jacob loved Rachel but was deceived by her father into sleeping with her older sister Leah. It was the custom for older sisters to marry before the younger ones. Ultimately Jacob did marry Rachel, but she at first was barren while her older sister bore children easily. Rachel therefore induced her servant Zilpah to have a baby for her by Jacob, another example of surrogacy. However, 'God remembered Rachel' later and she bore a son, Joseph. It was in bearing him that Rachel died, because she had great difficulty with the birth.

Contemporary knowledge of the role of semen in reproduction is demonstrated in the story of Onan, whose father was Judah. Onan 'spilled his seed upon the floor' by masturbation to prevent him fathering a child by his brother's wife as he had been ordered by Judah. His mother Tamar had twins in her womb and as she was giving birth a fetal hand appeared. The midwife tied a scarlet thread round the wrist to show which was the first born. This suggests that the first twin was a transverse lie, yet the hand was withdrawn so that birth was ultimately normal.

Exodus gives an early version of the Ten Commandments among which is 'You shall not covet your neighbour's wife'. There is concern here for the regulations of potentially disruptive relationships within society.

Leviticus gives instructions for purification after childbirth. Verse 12 says,

> 'A woman who becomes pregnant and gives birth to a son will be ceremonially unclean for seven days, just as she is unclean during her monthly period. On the eighth day the boy is to be circumcised. Then the woman must wait thirty-three days to be purified from her bleeding. She must not touch anything sacred or go to the sanctuary until the days of her purification are over. If she gives birth to a daughter, for two weeks the woman will be unclean, as in her period. Then she must wait sixty-six days to be purified from her bleeding.'

The cultural attitudes to women and their second-class citizenship are here vividly displayed. They have coloured the whole of subsequent western civilisation with its christian traditions. They made menstruation and childbirth shameful and to be hidden away.

Lessons to be learned from Old Testament teachings are:

1. Eve was responsible for the Fall of Man.
2. Women are cursed by the pains of childbirth.
3. Infertility is a disgrace. It may be offset by surrogacy.
4. Male homosexuality is abhorrent.
5. Female prostitution is accepted though frowned on.
6. Rape and bestiality are abhorrent.
7. Adultery is commonplace but sinful.
8. It is better to marry within the tribe rather than outside it.
9. Women are unclean at the time of menstruation and in the puerperium. The period of uncleanness is greater after the birth of a daughter than of a son.
10. Daughters are the possessions of their fathers, who may arrange their marriages.
11. Widows and orphans are to be protected.
12. Pregnancy late in life may be the subject of ridicule.

It is left to the reader to decide how many of these teachings are still accepted today, and how many may be relevant in determining the attitudes of modern societies. Some of the ideas expressed have been accepted, and some rejected by various societies and in different ages. But undoubtedly many of them remain significant and important to some. Each culture selects and rejects according to its own preconceptions.

CHAPTER THREE

Hellenistic and Roman Times (Soranus and Galen)

Alexander the Great (356–32 BC) of Macedon in his far-reaching campaigns carried elements of the Greek culture with him. His physician was Aristotle, whom some regard as the founder of science. As Greek, or Hellenic culture was absorbed by some of the conquered territories it was modified and came to be known to later historians as Hellenistic.

A main centre of this culture was Alexandria in Egypt. A medical school had become established there and at some time the Hippocratic library of Cos was moved to the city. Unfortunately most of it was destroyed in a fire started by christian zealots.

Two teachers in Alexandria, Erasistratus and Herophilus, both born about 303 BC, were able to study human anatomy because they were allowed to dissect the bodies of criminals. In many ancient and later cultures the body was looked upon as sacred and not to be defiled after death by dissection. But these two doctors made little contribution to the understanding of female pelvic anatomy. Following the Hellenistic period cultural dominance passed to the Roman Empire. It flourished, especially about the time of Christ. It boasted the first gynaecologist in known history – Soranus of Ephesus (AD 98–138). Ephesus was in Ionia, not far from the modern Turkish city of Smyrna (Izmir). It was then a major city and outpost of the Empire, and a great centre for trade with the East. It was the site of the Temple of Diana, the Huntress, who was also the goddess concerned with childbirth. Later, Soranus moved to Alexandria to the medical school. It was there that he probably learned something of the anatomy of the uterus, for his description of the organ suggests that he must have seen it at dissection.

Soranus' major work was *De arte Obstetrica Morbisque Mulierum* (On the art of obstetrics and the diseases of women). In this he described the uterus as being mobile within the pelvis and situated between the bladder and rectum. He knew it to be smaller in children and larger in those women who had had children. He knew of minor degrees of prolapse and the peritoneal coverings of the uterus. He measured the length of the vagina which he said was about 3–4" long.

In labour Soranus knew that the neck of the womb had to open up sufficiently widely to allow the baby to pass through. This means that he must have performed vaginal examinations. These were not otherwise commonly done by medical men. He thought that the ovaries were similar to testes and he confirmed the observation of Herophilus that the ovary had a suspensory ligament. He noted 'a certain sympathy between the uterus and the breasts' in knowing that they enlarged at puberty and during pregnancy and regressed in old age. He knew that the uterus was not essential to life for he cites instances in women and sows where the womb had been removed and the patients and animals survived. He had probably removed the uterus where it protruded from the vagina in extreme prolapse.

Soranus scotched the notion that the uterus was an animal which wandered far and wide in the body to cause symptoms of hysteria (NB. *globus hystericus*). Based on this belief was a treatment for prolapse, in which a woman stood astride a small fire burning unpleasant smelling substances designed to drive the animal back into its lair! Soranus advocated that midwives should have clean hands and be well-manicured.

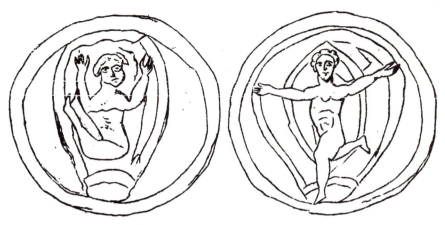

Fig. 3.1 'Fetus in utero' by Soranus

The girdle should be loosened in labour, which was an ancient belief. It was thought to be helpful in easing the pains of labour and hastening its progress. A warm hand on the abdomen in labour was comforting. Midwives were advised to explore the cavity of the uterus with the fingers after birth to extract blood clots and pieces of placenta. This potentially dangerous manoeuvre was practised for centuries and may have caused much loss of life due to infection carried in by the hand. The practice of feeling the cervix in labour, which he also advised, must also have caused infection on many occasions because there were no concepts of antisepsis and asepsis. In cases of severe bleeding after childbirth he packed the uterus with cloths, which must have been a prodigious feat in pre-anaesthetic days. It, too, was a technique practised for centuries, up to the present one.

Soranus gave instructions on how to treat the umbilical cord of the baby and its stump with dressings. In gynaecology he knew of fibroid tumours, vaginal examinations and speculum examinations of the cervix. From these last he knew of cancer of the cervix. He advocated the use of strips of lint inserted into the vagina to prevent conception. For massive prolapse he used half a pomegranate as a vaginal pessary.

From acquaintance with the Hippocratic canon Soranus knew of puerperal fevers and he used catheters to empty the bladder and to irrigate the uterus. He mistakenly believed that the bones of the pelvis separated during labour by the opening up of the symphysis pubis – a belief which persisted through many centuries. It meant that in difficult labour, and especially when there is obstruction caused by disproportion between the size of the baby's head and the pelvic cavity, the pelvis will enlarge to allow birth to occur. This, of course, is not so. Obstructed labour, when there are no artificial means to extract the baby, ultimately results in death of both baby and mother.

The major innovation of Soranus was the introduction and use of *internal version*. In this operation the baby is turned round within the uterus using a hand in the vagina and through the cervix. The head, which normally presents, even in an obstructed labour, is pushed up out of the pelvis by the operator's hand, a foot is sought and pulled down to emerge through the orifice of the vagina. It is quite impossible with the hand to find any purchase on the head so that it can never be withdrawn from the birth canal using the hands alone. But a leg is easy to grasp and can be pulled on quite hard to effect delivery in difficult cases. Bandages and even ropes can be tied to it too to increase pulling power.

Internal version was the only way to help a woman when her labour was obstructed by her bony pelvis being too small or her baby too large. It is probable that even after the successful prosecution of the operation in those ancient times the baby would have died, either before or after birth. Yet the mother's life might often have been saved by getting all the contents of the uterus out of her. To leave her on her own to cope with an obstructed labour was a sure way for both her and her baby to die.

Despite the obvious potential value of internal version as Soranus described it, it was ignored by doctors and midwives for about 14 centuries until Ambroise Paré of Paris rediscovered it. Its use after his time will be considered later.

Soranus moved to Rome, then becoming the centre of the civilised world, where *De Re Medicina* (Of Medical Matters) by Celsus had been published in 30 AD. It was especially remarkable for describing the four cardinal signs of inflammation – redness, swelling, heat and pain. Later centuries have added only loss of function. Though not a doctor Celsus advocated leaving illness to the *vis medicatrix naturae* – the healing force of nature. This was and is a helpful concept, for there is often a tendency on the part of helpers to indulge in meddlesome interference when leaving matters to nature might result in a better outcome. This is particularly true in midwifery where patience and careful observation of pregnant and labouring women are valuable attributes of midwives and obstetricians.

Shortly after him was Galen (AD c.131–201). He was primarily interested in medicine and surgery rather than midwifery, and was a most prolific writer. He had studied in Smyrna, near his birth place, as well as in Alexandria and Rome. He studied anatomy in animals because he maintained that the human body was the repository of the soul and therefore not to be defiled. This commended him and his writings to the church and this view held back the development of the basic science for medicine of human anatomy. Galen said that the uterus consisted of two horns, which is true of animals, but not of women. However, he assumed that women too had two horns to their uteri, and he said that male fetuses were carried in the right horn and female fetuses in the left. This notion keeps cropping up even today among the ignorant and it is entirely fallacious. However, one thing about which he was firm and correct was that it was not the fetus which initiated labour and forced its way into the outside world by its own efforts. He knew a great deal about other muscles and he was sure that the fetus was expelled by maternal factors of muscular contraction. This was another good idea which was lost for centuries.

Roman literature makes it certain that there were midwives and wise women concerned with pregnancy, labour and after. There were probably women doctors too, but they have left no permanent records of their practices, beliefs and teachings.

As before it should be noted that there were valuable insights into the understanding of matters of reproduction amid much nonsense. Most of the valuable observations were not even recognized as such at the time and did not get incorporated into practice, then or later. Perhaps this is not surprising since childbirth in all its aspects attracted little professional attention in the main, except by illiterates and those deemed to be of the inferior classes. Only very few outstanding practitioners left any kind of record behind them by which the state of the art and science of midwifery in Roman times may be judged now.

CHAPTER FOUR

The Renaissance of Learning

The Roman Empire declined. The works of Soranus were forgotten, but those of Galen flourished because they were acceptable to the medieval christian church. Christianity had gradually ousted most other religions within the boundaries of the Empire, which was far-flung. The clergy came to have much power and influence. They were well-educated, spoke and wrote the common language of Latin wherever they were in Europe and elsewhere. They often held high offices of state because of their educated superior abilities.

Yet the rising power of religion tended to stifle original thinking especially in what might have been perceived as science. The clergy had a monopoly of knowledge and controlled most forms of education. Their knowledge was not inclined to be innovative and questioning. They looked to the past in the Middle Ages movement of Scholasticism. They revered the old masters of antiquity and believed that little could be added to what they had taught and written. Because of this they happily preserved the works of ancient Greek civilisation, including those of Hippocrates. Nearer their own time they continued to rework and repeat the teachings of Galen. They were inclined to select him rather than others since he held to medical theories and practices in accord with their own religious beliefs. So the Middle Ages up to about 1500 were not conducive to many advances in medicine, and certainly not much in midwifery. Even the rise of the Arabian Empire, flourishing in the 7th and 8th centuries along both shores of the Mediterranean, and carrying the religion of Islam with it, as far as Spain from its centre in Baghdad, did not help the causes of women in childbirth. Both Christianity and Islam had little place for women in their very dominant religious cultures. Women were handmaidens for men and very definitely second-class citizens. With clergymen in power the teachings of the Bible and especially Genesis were enough to understand the place of women in christian society. They were all cast in the mould of Eve and therefore a constant and persistent reminder of temptation and evil. This was no climate of opinion in which great advances in the management of childbirth could be made. There was no reason why a celibate clergy should take any serious interest in the affairs of women, except to regulate them for the benefit of men.

Yet all was not totally black in these Dark Ages. The New Testament, too, had its place in cultural attitudes, 'Love thy neighbour as thyself' was a major commandment. Monastic foundations came to have infirmaria for the care of their sick monks, and they often took in ill travellers too, and lay people living nearby. There came therefore a tendency for some monks, or nuns in convents, to have a working knowledge of medicines, herbs and dressings and the elements of nursing. However they were as likely to invoke God to help in the healing processes as to seek physical remedies. Still there was no direct knowledge, understanding nor special care of childbearing women. This was true of both Western and Eastern christian Empires.

As with all cultures there were ideas arising within the medieval one which were destined to change its direction and modify its attitudes. The Arabian Empire disintegrated after the fall of Cordova in 1236. Mongols took Baghdad in 1258. The Turks sacked Constantinople in 1453 and dealt a severe blow to Orthodox Christianity thereby. These military conquests shook up cultures too and made them readier for change.

Salerno

An astonishing development for its time between the 9th and 12th centuries was the School of Salerno, on the west coast of Italy near Montecassino, where there was a Benedictine monastery. Legend has it that the School was founded by a Jew, an Arab, a Greek and a Roman. That is unlikely to be true but there is no doubt that Salerno was the recipient of ideas from all these cultures. This area including Sicily had been under the influences of all those civilisations over many centuries.

Salerno came under the patronage of kings and emperors. They required that the curriculum for medical education should be laid down and tested by examination by the masters and teachers of the school. Moreover before practising on their own, students or graduates had to remain under supervision for one year. This has a peculiarly modern ring. There were women physicians at Salerno. The most renowned was Trotula and she may have been a midwife as well as a doctor. A textbook of obstetrics of about 1050 is attributed to her, though it was probably not original but derived from older sources. It contained much on cosmetics.

Perhaps the most significant development at Salerno was the beginning of interest in anatomy. Human bodies could not be dissected for this was prohibited by Christianity and Islam. But there were dissections of pigs and at least this showed a willingness to test theory against facts, and not simply repeat the teachings of Galen. A book by Copho of the 11th century was called *Anatomia Porci*.

Church councils of 1130 and 1139 forbade clerics to practise medicine outside the walls of their institutions. This had the effect of increasing the laicisation of medicine. Lay medical practitioners were less hidebound by religious dogma than the clerics so that, in some ways, thinking and practice could become freer.

Adding to this freedom of thought was the founding of many universities from the 14th century onwards. Many of them had a medical faculty. It was not usually devoted purely to medicine but included the then developing sciences of all kinds, especially mathematics and astronomy. One such university was Montpellier in the south of France. It was well placed to be influenced both by the Arabian traditions from Cordova in Spain and the universities which had been founded in northern Italy at Bologna and Padua. After 1340 the dissection of executed criminals was allowed at Montpellier, and the practice was also known in Bologna where Mundinus was the first person to dissect a human female. However, even he described the uterus as consisting of two horns as Galen had done. It is, of course, just possible that his anatomical subject was one who did have the congenital abnormality of a bicornuate uterus.

Throughout the Middle Ages childbirth was professionally in the hands of midwives. They had virtually no formal education and were mostly illiterate. They were literally 'with-wives' which is the old meaning of the word 'midwife'. Many of these early midwives used birth stools for delivery. These were chairs with reclining backs and a large hole cut out of the seat – somewhat in the manner of a lavatory seat – from which the front portion had been removed. The woman sat on the horseshoe-shaped seat with her perineum over the cut-out. The midwife squatted or sat on the floor in front of her to receive the baby and the placenta into her lap. It was a system that had obvious merit for both mother and attendant. This was especially so since the whole area of the action was covered in clothes and cloths to keep everything hidden from sight as far as possible, for it was an immodest proceeding.

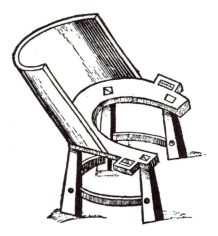

Fig. 4.1: An Obstetrical Chair

A special duty of the midwife was to baptise sickly babies as soon as possible. Sometimes the baptism was performed while the baby was still inside the woman. For this purpose there were special baptismal syringes. These were similar to enema syringes with a curved nozzle which could be inserted into the vagina. Water was then sprayed on the scalp of the baby while the holy incantations were made.

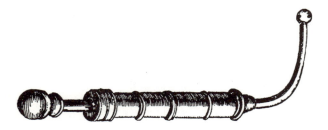

Fig. 4.2: A Baptismal Syringe

If labour was prolonged it was common to loosen the garments then lift the woman by her armpits and let her fall as heavily as possible as if to shake the baby out of the vagina. An alternative was to tie the woman to a ladder and then lift it up and bang it down on the floor several times.

Caesarean section

It is doubtful if this operation was performed much on the living woman during the Middle Ages, though sometimes it may have been done on a recently dead one. The *Lex Caesarea* of ancient Rome required that the fetus should be removed from a dead mother so that both might be separately buried, for religious reasons. Probably Julius Caesar was not born by caesarean section as myth sometimes suggests. The word 'caesarean' more probably derives from the Latin verb *'caedare'* meaning to cut. Each word of 'caesarean section' then means 'cut'.

The first recorded successful caesarean section was done in 1500 by Jacob Nüfer, a Swiss sow-gelder. He performed the operation on his wife when doctors had abandoned her to her inevitable fate. He must have had some knowledge of anatomy because of his trade and moreover he had the appropriate tools. Both mother and baby survived and she went on to produce other children.

There are cases, too, of self-inflicted caesarean sections. Girls conceiving out of wedlock were so ostracised by their communities and made to feel so ashamed that they were sometimes driven to deliver their babies abdominally and then dispose of them. It was an attempt to disprove the gossip about them. After such an horrific event one girl in Germany is recorded as having bound up her abdomen tightly and then walking five miles to try to show that she had never been pregnant. Later ages show that death for the mother is not an inevitable consequence of caesarean section. As many as 25 per cent may survive even without anaesthesia. The same is true of many major operations such as those of amputation, which was so frequently done.

Towards the end of the 16th century Scipione Mercurio (1540–1616), who studied in Bologna, published *La Commare o Riccoglitrice* in 1596. It was a book for midwives in which is described the position for labour with the patient's thighs hanging down over the edge of the bed so that the whole pelvis is rotated anteriorly. The intention was to make the labour easier by enlarging the inlet of the pelvis. It probably does not do this but it was taken up again by Gustav Adolf Walcher (1856–1935) of Germany in 1889. It became known as Walcher's position and was widely used. More interesting was that Mercurio described caesarean section, obviously on the living woman. He was however cautious about it, saying, 'before he puts his hand to work he must diligently consider whether there is another way of delivering the child beside this...'. He first counted the pulse and made an estimate of whether the woman was strong enough to withstand the operation. He described the preparation of the instruments, including a very sharp knife, sponges for mopping out the blood, the ligatures and needles for repairing the wound, the position of the patient sitting on the edge of the bed with her feet on the floor but lying well back or supported on cushions, and the dispositions of the strong, quiet assistants to hold the woman still.

The incision was to be marked out in ink avoiding an enlarged spleen or liver in the upper abdomen. The bladder at the lower end was also to be avoided, partly by having the midwife empty the bladder with a catheter. Ink marks were placed to show the site of sutures for repair of the abdominal wall. The vertical incision was to be made through the skin, fat, between the rectus muscles, through the peritoneum and down to the uterus. Strangely he advocated that the uterus should be cut transversely to avoid cutting into the testes, epididymis and spermatic vessels of the baby. The baby and placenta were to be delivered through the wounds, that in the abdomen being about six inches in length. Blood was to be mopped out of the abdominal cavity with the sponges and an assistant was to be ready to hand the sutures and needles to the surgeon, while he pressed on the intestines to keep them from extruding. A salve was to be applied to the wound. After the operation,

> 'The patient must live very quietly ... and eschew the use of wine at least for a fortnight, lest it produce inflammation; and the woman must keep indoors, where air does not harm her, and in short let her govern herself with as much diligence as would be occasioned by a body whose abdomen had suffered a mortal injury. This is enough about this new method of aiding difficult deliveries to help miserable patients.' (Quotations taken from *Classical Contributions to Obstetrics and Gynaecology* by Herbert Thoms, published by Charles C. Thomas, Springfield, Ill., 1935, p.105.)

Anatomically, of course, the operation is not difficult, but the interest here lies in the fact that Mercurio expected at least some of his patients to survive. He recognized too that sometimes there was nothing to help women in obstructed labour except this dire proceeding. He perpetuates the ancient belief that air is a cause of infection.

A textbook for midwives

In 1513 Eucharius Rösslin, a physician at Wörms in Germany, and later of Frankfurt, published a book called *Der Schwangern Frawen und Hebammen Roszgarten* (Rosegarden of Pregnant Women and Midwives). It became universally known as 'The Rosegarden'. It was written in vernacular German for the benefit of midwives but was later translated into Latin for wider dissemination.

Frankfurt was remarkable because a private benefaction of the 15th century had provided the city with municipal midwives, of whom there were ultimately five. This example was followed in several other German cities. Moreover the benefaction led to the appointment of a town physician, a post to which Rösslin was elected in 1506. One of his tasks was to license midwives to practise. He obviously took his duties very seriously, for it was his supervision of midwives that led to him writing his book, mainly for midwives.

Rösslin acknowledged debts to Hippocrates and Galen, but it is especially interesting that he took much of his material from Moschion, who had translated the works of Soranus into Latin. Even then, however, the operation of internal podalic version was not taken up and used.

'The Rosegarden' was called *De Partu Hominis* in Latin. It was translated into English by Richard Jonas who called it *The Byrthe of Mankind*. It was published in 1540 by Thomas Raynalde, probably in the churchyard of St Paul's Cathedral. Sometimes it was called 'The Woman's Boke'. It was enormously successful. The last print in English appeared in 1676 and in German in 1730, and by then it had gone through 40 editions.

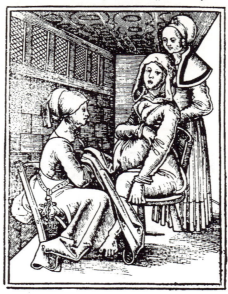

Fig. 4.3: Frontispiece of 'Der Swangeren Frauen und Hebammen Rosengarten'

It was remarkably influential in the practice of midwifery. It was, in fact, the first book to deal with midwifery alone, not mixed up with medicine and surgery.

> The book contained a crude figure of the baby in a single-chambered uterus, nothing like as accurate as the later one of Leonardo's. The birth-stool was recommended and the midwife was to sit in front of the labouring woman and was advised to 'instruct and comfort the party, not only refreshing her with good meate and drink, but also with sweet words, giving her hope of a good speedie deliverance ... also stroking gently with her hands her belly about the Navell, for that helpeth to depress the birth downeward. But this must the midwife above all things take heede of, that she compell not the woman to labour before the birth come forward, and shew itself. For before that time, all labour is in vaine, labour as much as yee list. And in this case many times it cometh to passe, that the party hath laboured so sore before the time, that when she should labour indeed, her might and strength is spent before in vaine, so that shee is not now able to helpe herself, and that is a perilous case.' (From *Eternal Eve* by Harvey Graham, 1950, p. 144.)

This excellent advice is known to every modern trained midwife. Bearing down before full dilatation of the cervix causes swelling of its anterior lip and obstructs labour. In fact this sensible waiting practice derives ultimately from Hippocrates and Soranus. It is especially to be noted that the advice was directed to midwives. Almost never were doctors admitted to the rooms of labouring women. A Dr Wertt of Hamburg in 1552 entered a lying-in room dressed as a woman so that he could observe what happened. He was burned at the stake for such impropriety.

Jacob Rueff of Switzerland produced another textbook for midwives in 1554. It followed 'The Rosegarden' in nearly every particular. It was called *De Conceptu et Generatione Hominis* (The Conception and Generation of Mankind). It contained a chapter on monsters, or deformed babies. These were deemed to be the result of the woman consorting with the Devil. This was a terrible sentence to pass on these poor women in those bigoted times.

In one famous picture of Rueff's there are astrologers in the background casting the newborn baby's horoscope.

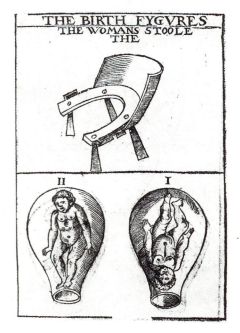

Fig. 4.4: Frontispiece of 'De Conceptu et Generatione Hominis'

Anatomy

Perhaps the outstanding scientific achievement of the Renaissance was the rise of anatomy as the subject basic to the practice of all medicine and surgery and midwifery. A landmark was the publication in 1543 of *De Humani Corporis Fabrica* (On the fabric of the Human Body). It was by Andreas Vesalius (1514–1564), a Belgian who was Professor of Anatomy at Padua in northern Italy. The originality of the book was that it was firmly based in practical dissections done by Vesalius himself. The dissections were depicted by competent artists. There was no idle repetition of what Galen and other ancients had written. He refuted Galen by showing that the uterus was a single-chambered organ. For its time it was an astonishing departure from customary repetitive book-based teaching.

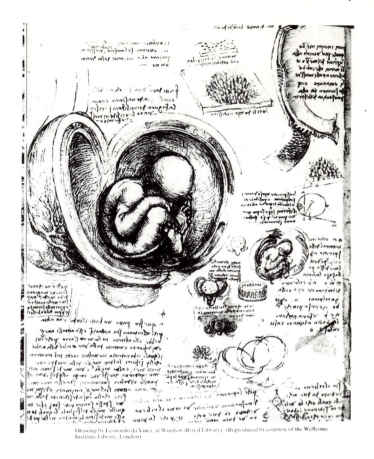

Drawing by Leonardo da Vinci, at Windsor (Royal Library). (Reproduced by courtesy of the Wellcome Institute Library, London)

Fig. 4.5: 'Fetus in Utero' by Leonardo Da Vinci

Yet artists already knew much anatomy. Leonardo da Vinci (1452–1519) produced some wonderful drawings and paintings of many parts of the human body. The one most relevant here is that of the fetus within the uterus. It is beautiful in its own right, but it is anatomically exceedingly accurate. But there seems to have been little rapport between art and science then, a division which has tended to remain.

There was some increasing interest in female anatomy. Gabriele Falloppio (1523–1562) was a pupil of Vesalius, ultimately following him as Professor of Anatomy at Padua. It is well-known that he described the Fallopian tube, but he also wrote of the ovaries, uterus, round ligaments, the clitoris and the hymen. He knew of the ovarian and uterine arteries but had no idea of their functions. He disposed of the idea that the ovaries were like testes. He had cut into them and seen that they contained little vesicles, quite unlike the cross section of a testis. It was Falloppio who named the vagina (a sheath) and the placenta (a cake), terms which have been used ever since. All these findings were recorded in his *Observationes Anatomicae* (Observations in Anatomy) published in Venice in 1561.

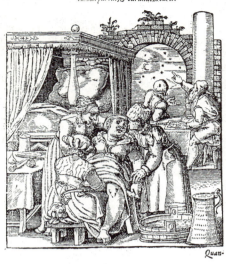

LIBER
LIBER QVARTVS.
DE VARIETATIBVS NON NA-
turalis partus, & earundem curis.

Quan-

Fig. 4.6: Frontispiece from 'The Byrth of Mankind'

Syphilis

The year after Falloppio died his book *De Morbo Gallico* (On the French Disease) was published. This dealt with the newly introduced disease now known as syphilis. It had probably been brought to Europe by sailors returning from North America which had been discovered by Christopher Columbus in 1492. It may have been endemic among the Indian tribes there. On introduction to Europe it raged rapidly through the populations, and the disease was much more acute then than it is now. Death from the disease occurred in a very few years, rather than over as many as 20 years or more in the mid-20th century, before a cure was found. Many infectious diseases show the same pattern in that when introduced to a susceptible community the disease can be very acute and have a high mortality. Over many years such communities may develop a degree of immunity so that the disease becomes more chronic and slower in producing its ill-effects. This may be happening now in HIV (human immunovirus) infections, where the time from infection to the development of AIDS (acquired immunodeficiency syndrome) seems to be increasing. Originally it was about one to two years and is now nearer ten in many instances.

On first introduction of syphilis it was called the 'Spanish disease' by the French and the 'French disease' by the Spaniards and Italians. Every country attributed it to some other one. The disease of syphilis was so named after the shepherd Syphilus. He was the subject of a poem called *Syphilis sive morbus gallicus* (Syphilis or the French disease) by Girolamo Fracastorio (1478–1553), also known as Fracastorius. It was published in Venice in 1530. Syphilus was infected and the poem describes his symptoms and notes that the disease is a venereal one. Fracastorius recommended the use of mercury in treatment and this remained in vogue up to the middle of the 20th century. However, Falloppio opposed its use, probably correctly. It was not until much later that syphilis in pregnancy was recognized as a potent cause of stillbirth, neonatal death and sickly children. Other anatomists, based mainly in northern Italy, wrote on various aspects of their subject. One of them was Matteo Realdo Colombo (1516–1559) who wrote on the pulmonary circulation and described the valves in the heart. Fabricius ab Acquapendente (1533–1619) described the valves in veins and probably influenced William Harvey in his discovery of the circulation of the blood, since Harvey visited Padua at the time when Fabricius was working there. He was also interested in embryology. In 1600 he published *De formatio foetu* (The Formation of the Foetus). This, too, may have influenced Harvey, who wrote on the same subject and had great influence on the development of midwifery in England.

Contracted pelvis and disproportion

Another anatomist interested in embryology was Giulio Cesare Aranzi (1530–1589) also known as Arantius. He wrote about it in his book of 1564, *De Humano foetu* (Of the Human Foetus). But more important for modern midwifery is that he described small and deformed bony pelves as causes of difficult and obstructed labour.

> 'If, however the pubic bones, due to the fault of the formative faculty, have not been favourably arranged, that is to say if they are too broad and in the exterior region so compressed that they become humped rather than concave on the inside, and if they come very near the sacrum and coccyx then the parts of the parturient become so narrow that the road is not wide enough for the foetus, even if turned upon its head according to nature, especially if it is endowed with a relatively large and solid head ... And, what is worse the helping hand of the operator which is about to bring aid, cannot reach there because of the narrowness of the parts. Thus it usually happens that not only the foetus but the puerpera herself succumbs; sometimes also necessity herself compels the extraction of the child, which is already dead and putrescent, with difficulty and piece by piece.' (From *Eternal Eve* by Harvey Graham, 1950, p.162).

There are hints in this extract that he might have been describing a rachitic pelvis, with the pubic bones pushed inwards and the brim of the pelvis flattened. There is a hint, too, of the use of internal podalic version in the reference to the hand bringing aid. The extraction of the dead fetus in pieces by the use of hooks and other instruments was known.

Ergot

In 1596 the physicians of Marburg, a town about 50 miles north of Frankfurt, investigated a disease called St Anthony's Fire. Those who suffered from it felt intense burning sensations in the skin and developed gangrene of the fingers and toes and sometimes larger parts of limbs, which sometimes simply fell off. There were abdominal symptoms too of cramping pains due to gut contractions. The uterus also contracted often giving rise to pain and abortion or premature labour.

The cause of the disease was found to be the ingestion of a black fungus infesting rye – *Claviceps purpurea*. This was called ergot. It only affected crops in wet and cold weather. Such contaminated rye was discarded when there was a good harvest, but had to be used for making bread when harvests were poor. It is highly likely that many midwives already knew of these properties of ergot and used the fungal grains to bring about abortions, or labour, or to hasten labour.

Another effect of eating contaminated rye was the 'dancing sickness'. The people who had eaten it went into a kind of frenzy, dancing and prancing for hours on end. The cause was LSD or ∂-lysergic acid, also present in the fungus, and a most powerful hallucinogen, often much abused in the mid-20th century.

Internal podalic version

This was the major clinical advance in midwifery in the 16th century. It was a revival of the operation, first described by Soranus of Ephesus in the second century AD, by Ambroise Paré (1510–1590) of Paris. He was the outstanding French surgeon of his day and made many contributions to civil and military surgery. He was carefully conservative and introduced ligatures again for the control of haemorrhage in amputations. He dressed wounds with gentle salves rather than hot pitch which had been the widely used method. His philosophy was summed up in his famous saying: '*Je le pansait; Dieu le guarit*' (I dressed him; God healed him).

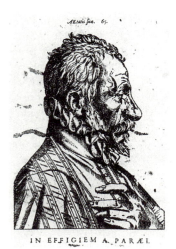

Fig. 4.7: Portrait of Ambroise Paré

When labour was not progressing Paré described how the woman should be suitably, yet gently, trussed to hold her heels against her buttocks, with knees and hips flexed, and with helpers to separate her knees to allow the operator access to the genital tract. The baby's head was to be pushed up to the upper part of the uterus. A foot was to be sought by the fingers and pulled out to the exterior and then drawn upon further. The hands had to be clean and the nails pared. All parts were to be abundantly treated with warm oil, and they had to be covered to preserve decency.

Paré wrote of the operation,

'and so turn him that his feet may come forwards, and when hee hath brought his feet forwards, hee must draw one of them gently out at the neck of the womb, and then hee must binde it with som broad and soft silken band a little above the heel with an indifferent slick [slip] knot, and when hee hath so bound it, he must put it up again into the womb, then he must put his hand in again, and finde out the other foot, and draw it also out of the womb, and when it is out of the womb, let him draw out the other again whereunto hee had before tied the one end of the band, and when hee hath them both out, let him join them both together, and so by little and little let him draw all the whole bodie from the womb. Also other women or Midwives may help the endeavor of the Chirurgian [surgeon], by pressing the patient's bellie with their hands downwards as the infant goeth out: and the woman herself by holding her breath, and closeing her mouth and nostrils, and by driveing downwards with great violence, may verie much help the expulsion...'
(*Classical Contributions to Obstetrics and Gynaecology*, by Herbert Thoms. Published by Chas. C. Thomas, 1935, p.101).

Paré went on further to describe how to deal with the arms and how it might be necessary to insert a hook into the mouth or eye-socket and pull on it if there should be further delay in delivery, which otherwise could not be overcome. It was gruesome but the alternative was to allow the mother to die, the baby probably being already dead. This description was published in 1549 with the title, *Briefve collection de l'administration anatomique: avec la maniere de conjoindre les os: et d'extraire les enfants tant mors que vivant du ventre de la mere, lors que nature de soy ne peult venir a son effect* (Brief collection of anatomical exercises: with the manner of union of the bones: and the extraction of infants more dead than alive from the abdomen of the mother, when nature of itself cannot bring about this effect).

He made an error which misled him and many subsequent generations, because of his immense and deserved authority. He thought that the cavity of the pelvis enlarged in labour by slackening of its joints, opening up the symphysis pubis and the sacro-iliacs. He came to this conclusion after dissecting a woman recently hanged a few weeks after the birth of her baby. It may be that by chance he had lighted on a woman with pelvic osteoarthropathy in which there is an almost pathological separation of the bones. That only occurs very rarely. The importance of the mistake was that labours were often allowed to proceed overlong in the hope that the pelvis would enlarge to allow the baby through. Such inordinate delay, based on this false premise, could be disastrous.

The 15th and 16th centuries, roughly the period of the Renaissance, show that some of the foundations of midwifery were being slotted into place. The beginnings of scientific anatomy made some progress in understanding the structure of the female bony pelvis and its contents. Instruction and regulation of midwives was beginning. The essence was gentle conservative watching over labour. Although not widely enjoined, the operations of internal podalic version and even, in extreme cases, caesarean section could occasionally be performed with some success to help women out of their difficult labours. Those would otherwise have killed them. The practice of removing the dead fetus piecemeal, with hooks and other instruments, when it was dead had to be used, also to save the mother's life.

There was then no antenatal care nor any understanding of pregnancy and its complications. Fits seem to have been accepted as not worthy of comment. Haemorrhages must have been awful, uncomprehended and leading to therapeutic impotence on the part of helpers. Yet a start had been made on building the modern edifice of midwifery.

CHAPTER FIVE

Seventeenth Century: The Handy Operation

Padua still shone brightly in the scientific world early in this century. Galileo Galilei (1564–1642) was using both a telescope and a microscope there in 1610. The microscope had been invented a little earlier in Holland by Zacharias Jansen (fl. 1590) It was then very crude, with just two lenses, and difficult to use, but in later times it opened up a whole new world of biology and medicine. It was Galileo who said that 'The Book of Nature is written in mathematical characters'. It is a principle which has guided the development of science ever since. Measurement and mathematics are the very basis of all sciences.

At about the same time as Galileo, Sanctorius of Padua invented a clinical thermometer, although temperature measurement was not widely adopted in medicine until much later. He also began the study of physiology by constructing a balance in which he was weighed regularly. He showed that if he took nothing by mouth he lost weight, which he correctly believed was due to loss of water and this he called 'invisible perspiration', still to be allowed for in fluid balance charts.

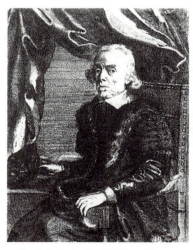

Fig. 5.1: Portrait of William Harvey

William Harvey (1578–1657), the great English physician and discoverer of the circulation of the blood, was a student in Padua where he learned of the valves in veins from Fabricius ab Acquapendente, and perhaps of the pulmonary circulation. He was probably also stimulated to take an interest in the development of the fetus by the work of Fabricius. Apart from his *De Motu Cordis et Sanguinis in Animalibus* (On the motion of the heart and blood in animals) of 1628, he also wrote *De Generatione Animalium* (On the Generation of Animals) in 1651. This book had a chapter on *De Partu* (birth) which described the processes of birth and how they should be managed. It was very influential and subsequent generations have called him the 'Father of British Midwifery'.

As regards embryology Harvey described his meticulous observations on chick embryos. As a result of these he subscribed to the theory of Epigenesis, in opposition to the theory of Preformation. Preformationists believed that at fertilisation all organs were already in being and simply had to grow. The Epigeneticists believed that male and female semen blended and that out of this mixture there had first to be differentiation of the organs to be followed later by growth in size. This is essentially the correct view.

Textbooks for midwives

In 1609 Jacques Guillemau (1550–1613) a pupil of Paré's published *L'Heureux Accouchement des Femmes* (The Happy Delivery of Women). Its purpose was to instruct midwives on the basis of Paré's teachings. However the majority of midwives of the time were unable to read or write. All too often they were ignorant and self-opinionated and must often have wreaked havoc on their patients. Yet there were signs that a slow change in their education and training was beginning.

A remarkable book, also of 1609, was written by the midwife Louise Bourgeois (1563–1636). It was called *Observations Diverses sur la Sterilite, Perte de Fruict, Foecundite, Accouchements, et Maladies des Femmes, et Enfants Nouveaux Naiz* (Diverse observations on sterility, loss of fruit [presumably miscarriage], fecundity, childbirth, and diseases of women, and newborn infants). It was translated into English in 1659 when it was called 'Compleat Midwives' Practice Enlarged'. The work was also based on Paré's teaching which included rupturing the membranes to induce premature labour. It is to be noted that these books were written in the vernacular and not in Latin.

Louise Bourgeois was unusual in that she was a product of the Hôtel Dieu in Paris, from where she became a licensed midwife of the city. She was obviously well-educated and trained, as well as having high social standing. In 1601 she delivered Marie de Medici of the Dauphin, who became Louis XIII. So there were a few literate midwives, there was some training for them at the Hôtel Dieu and there was some licensing and regulation of them, at least in France.

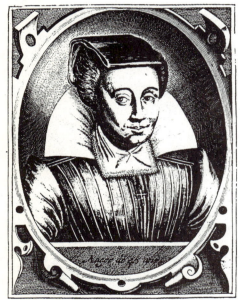

En ce parfait tableau le defaut de peinture
Se connoist aujourdhuy clairement a nos yeux
Pource qu'on n'y peut veoir que du corps la figure
Non l'esprit admiré pour chef d'oeuure des cieux
S. Hacquin.

Figure 5. 2: Portrait of Louise Bourgeois

There were moves in England, too, to regulate the practice of midwives. Peter Chamberlen II (of whom more later) suggested to James I in 1616 that midwives should be licensed. He was not entirely altruistic since he wished to head any regulatory body himself and make some money out of it. Peter Chamberlen III returned to the same charge in 1634, when he advocated that a corporation under the Royal College of Physicians should train and license midwives. He, too, expected to head such a venture. He went so far as to insist that two midwives, Mrs Shaw and Mrs Whipp, should meet him monthly to be instructed in the art of midwifery. They complained about this and as result Chamberlen was reprimanded by a bishop's enquiry. It was then required that all doctors and midwives in London should be licensed by the bishop.

Doctors, too, were slowly coming under some formalisation of training and licensing. The Royal College of Physicians was founded in 1518, the Company of Barber-Surgeons in 1540 and the Society of Apothecaries in 1617. The beginnings of the separation into physicians, surgeons and general practitioners can be seen in these foundations. There was yet no formal room for man-midwives, as they came to be called. In fact the Royal College of Physicians forbade any of its licentiates to practise midwifery. If midwives required medical help they had to call in a barber-surgeon or an apothecary.

A further textbook from France was that by the famous François Mauriceau (1637–1709). It was published in Paris in 1668 and was called *Des Maladies des Femmes Grosses et Accouchées* (some maladies of women pregnant and brought to childbed). It was the outstanding work of its time. After a description of the female genital organs it is divided into three parts, dealing in turn with pregnancy, labour, the puerperium and the newborn. It is a format which has been almost universally adopted by later textbooks of midwifery and obstetrics.

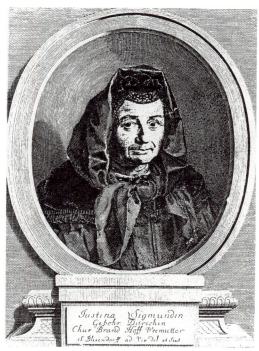

Fig. 5.3: Portrait of Justine Siegemundin

In 1671 there was the English book by Jane Sharp entitled *The Midwives Book* which later became called the 'Compleat Midwife's Companion'. Another midwife, Justine Siegemundin (1650–1705), lived in Germany and was celebrated as the 'pious Justine', because of her frequent references to God. Her book, in German, was published in 1690. She was responsible for the introduction of rupture of the membranes in an attempt to control antepartum bleeding. She was Court Midwife to Frederick III of Prussia. The book was written in question and answer form between Justine and Christina, whom she was instructing. The name of 'accoucheur' was first bestowed on Jules Clément by Louis XIV in 1663. The accolade was given after Clément had delivered the king's mistress, the Marquise de Montespan.

Clinical practice

The best insight into practice of this time is provided by Percivall Willughby (1596–1685) in his *Observations in Midwifery*. To this was appended a partial summary of the main work called 'The Countrey Midwifes Opusculum' or *Vade Mecum*. Both parts were intended for the instruction of midwives. He described his practice from about 1640 to 1670 based on his notes of about 150 cases he had attended. Unfortunately it was not printed in his own time, although it seems to have been fairly widely known.

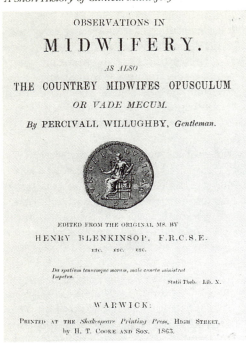

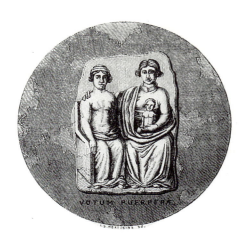

Fig. 5.4: First and title pages from 'Observations in Midwifery'

Surprisingly it was first printed in Dutch from Leyden in 1724. It was not finally printed in English until 1863 when Willughby's original manuscripts were edited by Henry Blenkinsop F.R.C.S.E.

Willughby tried to obtain a formal education in medicine but his finances ran out. He therefore became apprenticed to a Mr van Otten of London, who was licensed by the Barber-Surgeons. He died in 1624 shortly after Willughby had joined him, so he went into practice in Derby, not far from his original home. He became an Extra-Licentiate of the Royal College of Physicians in 1640–41. This was the qualification granted to those who practised outside London, after an examination. Willughby based his book on his own experience, though he had read the literature on midwifery widely. He particularly revered William Harvey, and quoted him on 16 occasions. Harvey was his friend and Willughby was visited by him. He wrote:

> 'I know none but Dr Harvey's directions and method, the which I wish all midwives to observe and follow and oft to read over and over again; and in so doing they will better observe, understand, and remember the sayings and doings of that most worthy, good, and learned Doctor whose memory ought to be had for ever in great esteem with midwives and child-bearing women.'

So Willughby exemplified the best practice of his times. He knew the signs of the onset of labour, and he attributed that to the baby being short of food. He advised against rupturing the membranes artificially and in that he opposed both Paré and Louise Bourgeois. However they only did this when they thought that the baby was too big to pass through the pelvis.

Willughby advocated that a woman in early labour should be given an enema and her bladder should be emptied by catheter if that was necessary. The enema was to consist of about 6 fluid ounces and was to be held as long as possible before evacuation. This was intended to help the onset of proper labour, for he recognized spurious labour in which painful uterine contractions which do not dilate the cervix can be misleading.

Willughby firmly upbraided many midwives and their practices. He condemned those who 'haled' [hauled] the woman to the obstetric stool at the first signs of labour. It seems that they would then spend much time and effort in manually dilating the cervix and stretching the vagina and perineum using oils, butter and lard for lubrication. Often they would rupture the membranes too. Because of these practices he recommended that the obstetric stool should be abandoned and the woman should instead lie on her bed or a pallet, so hoping to keep officious meddling midwives at bay.

In 1656 he was called by a countryman to his wife, about four miles out of the city.

> '[There] I found this woman sitting up, and very faint, and her young midwife troublesome, and sharply chiding the woman in pain, telling her, That shee could have found in her heart to have tied her feet in her chaire, and so, whether shee would or not, to have delivered her. I gave the woman and the midwife good words ... I leave all women to their liberty to make choice of their midwife, yet I will not bee forward to perswade them to take such a midwife, as will bind them, perforce, fast in their chaires, against their wills. Or, that will pull, stretch or hale their bodies, or use any violence to enforce the womb, in hopes of a speedier delivery. Such strugglings and doings make a difficult, painfull, and long labour.'

Regrettably there are many other such passages in the *Observations*. He instances several cases of women who delivered easily and safely without assistance from anyone, when they were on journeys or had no time to call a midwife. On this knowledge he based his counsel of non-interference when matters were proceeding normally.

Willughby particularly condemned the notion, then prevalent among midwives, that difficult labour was due to the 'baby sticking to the back'. This led some of them to put their hands right inside the uterus to sweep the baby away from the uterine wall to unstick it. So meddlesome were some of them that he records a case of a midwife pulling and tugging away at a cancer which she had not recognized as such, believing the woman to be in labour when she was not even pregnant.

Willughby thought the best position for delivery was for the woman, on her bed, to kneel on a firm bolster with the feathers shaken down to one end. Her knees were to be slightly apart and the midwife was to kneel in front of her so that she could put her arms round the neck of her assistant or on her shoulders. The midwife could help in drawing out the baby but there was no need to guard the perineum for that was supported by the soft bolster. 'The midwife's office, or duty, in a naturall birth, is no more, but to receive the child, and afterwards to fetch the after-birth if need require.'

It was common then to remove the placenta manually after every birth, but Willughby only wanted this to be done 'if need require'. If there was difficulty in delivering the shoulders the advice was for the woman to take up the knee–chest position. The assistant then approaching from the rear had a better chance of effecting delivery more easily, by moving the head up and down, till one shoulder emerged.

The handy operation

Willughby's answer to virtually every serious problem in cephalic delivery or transverse lie was internal podalic version, which he called 'the handy operation'. If the breech was presenting he made no effort to turn the baby as many midwives did by pummelling and pushing on the mother's abdomen or even attempting internal cephalic version. On one occasion he was appalled that midwives tossed a woman in a blanket in an effort to make the baby turn round. He was very sure that the pubic bones did not separate in labour, and so refuted both Harvey and Paré. So when the labour was obstructed there was no point in waiting further. To perform the version he had the woman in the knee–chest position, with her bottom as high in the air as possible. This might, by gravity, help to get the head out of the pelvis. With the head high above the pelvic brim he advocated that a hand should be inserted into the uterus to seek a foot and pull it down with the fingers. When this was done the same procedure was to be carried out with the other foot. He described how the foot could be distinguished from a hand by the heel and by not being able to abduct the big toe, as the thumb can be widely abducted from the main body of the hand.

With the feet drawn down the woman was to straighten up somewhat so that the weight of the baby would aid delivery. A cloth round the legs and buttocks of the baby improved the grip of the operator. If the arms were extended alongside the head, one was to be hooked out with a finger. Then the body was to be rotated so that the face pointed towards the rear of the mother. A finger in the mouth helped to keep the baby's head flexed. This, in fact, was what came to be known in the next century as the Mauriceau-Smellie-Veit manoeuvre in breech delivery.

When the 'handy operation' failed, as it sometimes did, even in Willughby's hands, then he had to have recourse to the hook or crotchet, this being a firm blunt hook with a handle. It had to be inserted carefully, preferably with a hand protecting the maternal tissues. It was then rotated so as to catch on some part of the baby, e.g. the chin, the mouth, the eye socket, or it might be driven into the skull. The baby, of course, would already be dead but the force necessary to effect delivery must often have seriously damaged the mother. But the alternative would have been to let her die of exhaustion.

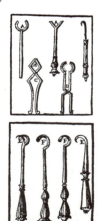

All too often Willughby was called in to deal with a hand which the midwife had pulled down out of the vagina. This is especially liable to happen when there

Fig. 5.5: Hooks or crotchets from 'La Commare o Riccoglitrice'

is a transverse lie, when the baby is crosswise over the inlet of the bony pelvis. He often found that the woman was bruised all about her perineum and vagina as a result of violent manipulations, and the tugging and pulling by the midwife. The arm was bruised and swollen too. On a few occasions he found that the midwife had cut the arm off and was plunging thatcher's hooks and knives into the baby's body. There were cases too where midwives cut into the head, quartering it, so that the brain matter was extruded and the skull collapsed. This last may not be quite as bad as it at first sounds. Perforation of the skull in otherwise insuperable obstruction was much used by later obstetricians when the baby was dead.

Willughby described fits occurring in pregnancy but knew he could do nothing about them. He also knew of the 'white leg' complicating the puerperium though he had no idea of its cause, now known to be deep venous thrombosis. Abscesses sometimes discharged from the pelvis but he had no idea of the cause of these except 'putrefaction'. Birth trauma causing fistulae between bladder and/or rectum and vagina he observed but knew that attempts to repair them often failed. The result of these traumas was a life of misery and seclusion for the unfortunate women, for there was no control of bladder or bowel.

He was greatly perturbed by haemorrhages before birth. Presciently he wrote, 'still I conceive that the cause of flouding is the separating of some part of the after-birth from the sides of the womb ...' Again with great insight he knew that the answer to flooding was that, 'it is delivery and only delivery that must do the deed'. He was so perturbed by bleeding that he prayed,

> 'If possible, I heartily could wish that some worthy practitioner would bee pleased to direct some powerfull wayes, or medicines, to bridle this raging, destroying evil. Women would have cause to acknowledge his worth, and all succeeding ages would give him thanks.'

It must have been appalling to witness such antepartum haemorrhage knowing that nothing could be done about it except stand helplessly by as life expired.

Willughby knew of fetal death in utero and that sometimes it led to what later became known as maceration. But he had found that sometimes when a midwife declared the baby to be dead he was able to show that there was still pulsation in the umbilical cord or that the hand of the baby gripped his finger. He described cases of phantom pregnancy. Its importance was that if the midwife was deceived into thinking the woman was pregnant she might start massaging the vagina and trying to force the cervix open. Caesarean section he would have nothing to do with,

> 'for the Caesarean section I do not like it. It hath proved unfortunate to severall, under whose hands the women have perished, and it is not used in England. Dr James Primrose holdeth it to bee a rash piece of work, and to do it in a living woman, a practice to be abhorred.'

> 'And to conclude, it is my opinion, That, in all difficult and crosse [transverse lie] births, The only way, and the *ultimum refugium* [ultimate refuge] to save

the mother, and the child, is, not to reduce the birth to the head, but to draw it forth by the feet, which may quickly, and easily, with safety, bee performed.'

It is to be remembered that this was advice to midwives, who when occasion demanded were to perform this operation. There were certainly not enough doctors then to cope with the problems of difficult labour.

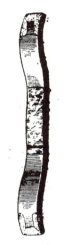

Fig. 5.6: Lever

The only other method that was sometimes used by others in this century was the lever. This was simply a curved metal band, about 12 inches long and one inch wide, which was slipped up over the baby's head when it was low down in the pelvis. The intention was then to lever the baby's head out using the symphysis pubis as a fulcrum. It may have worked on occasions but was liable to cause much damage to the soft parts of the vagina and urethra.

Another instrument was the speculum matricis. It was usually a three-bladed speculum which could be inserted into the cervix and then by a screw device the blades could be forced apart to open the cervix. It never had much vogue. In 1671 James Woolveridge published *Speculum Matricis*, or 'The Expert Midwives' Handmaid, Catechistically Composed', which means that it was in question and answer form.

Willughby made a plea for post-mortem examinations to be done. At an autopsy he had seen an intra-abdominal pregnancy, i.e. outside the uterus and in the peritoneal cavity. He regretted that they were not normally performed in England but

'In France, and the Low Countries, they have many privileges, and customs which we cannot obtain in England. They open dead bodies, without any mutterings of their friends. Should one of us desire such a thing, an odium of inhumane cruelty would bee upon us by the vulgar and common people.'

There is no doubt that people could be cruel and unkind. Punishments were often harsh. Willughby cites the case of a simple girl who did not know she was pregnant. In the middle of the night she arose from between her two companions in bed and went to a nearby stream to ease her belly-ache. There she delivered she knew not what and left it there. But

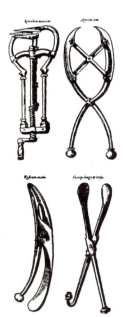

Fig. 5.7: Speculum matricis from 'De Conceptu et Generatione Hominis'

her two bedfellows had followed her and they found a dead baby. She was brought before the court where Willughby interceded for her. But 'The judg, nor jury, regarded her simplicity. They founnd her guilty, the judg condemned her, and shee was, afterwards, hanged for not having a woman by her, at her delivery.' It seems that this was the law of the time. However, if the baby had been born alive and she had suckled it at the breast, this poor 'foole' of a girl might have been spared.

On another occasion a young woman was seen by some soldiers of the Civil War to bury her dead baby under some feathers in a farm outhouse. The soldiers intimidated the court and,

> 'the Jury would not find her guilty of murder, for that shee was an handsome, comely creature, and beloved of the souldiers, that then pitied her misfortunes. For which reason John Shaw, the foreman of the Jury, pitying the woman, and willing to ingratiate the souldiers to bee his friends, would not find her guilty, and said, hee thought it no reason that a woman should be hanged for a mistaken harsh word or two in the Statute. The Souldiers smiled and rejoyced at her delivery. But some of the Derby Magistrates frowned, and were offended, but they durst not shew, or utter their thoughts in words, or deeds, for the cause aforementioned.'

One might be permitted to wonder if one of the soldiers was the father of the infant!

The obstetric forceps, one of the great advances in clinical midwifery had been invented towards the end of the 17th century, but it was kept as a family secret by the Chamberlens. The instrument only came into more general use in the 18th century, so its story will be taken up in the next chapter.

There was some scientific advance of relevance to midwifery. Jan Swammerdam (1637–1680) in Holland showed that the lungs of a newborn baby who had breathed would float in water, whereas those of a stillborn would not. He saw red blood corpuscles under the microscope too. Regnio de Graaf (1641–1673), also in Amsterdam, saw human ova and described the follicles in the ovary which contained them. They have been known as Graafian follicles ever since. The work was published in 1672 as *De Mulierum Organis Generationi Inservientibus* (On the organs serving generation in women). It followed a work of 1668 in which he had described the generative organs in men.

A pupil of Swammerdam's was Caspar Bartholin secundus (1655–1738), who, in 1678, described the glands at the rear of the vulva, which have borne his name since. He exploded the notion of there being female semen. He showed that discharge came from the cervix, vagina and the vulval glands and not from the ovaries. Another contribution from Amsterdam was that of Antony van Leeuwenhoek (1632–1723) who described spermatozoa he had seen under the microscope in 1679, and in 1683 he saw bacteria too. Earlier still Robert Hooke (1635–1703) in England had seen bacteria in 1665 and gave the name of cells to those basic structures in his book *Micrographia*. These were all astonishing observations made without the benefit of staining techniques.

Vital statistics, which became so important in measuring progress in midwifery began in 1662. John Graunt (1620–1674) of London in 1662 produced *Natural and Political Observations mentioned in a following index, and made upon the Bills of Mortality, London.* He was a friend of Sir William Petty (1623–1687) who published *Political Arithmetic* in 1683 and *Several Essays in Political Arithmetic* in 1699.

One of the great landmarks of scientific history was published in 1687. It was the 'Principia Mathematica' of Isaac Newton (1642–1727). Its full name was *Philosophiae Naturalis Principia Mathematica* (Mathematical Principles of Natural Philosophy). It had profound influence at the time and that still continues, especially in physics and astronomy but also in other sciences. The changed attitudes to science exemplified by this work have had many later effects in midwifery and medicine.

CHAPTER SIX

Seventeenth Century: Obstetric Forceps

The problem with delivering a baby presenting by the breech, or lying tranversely across the brim of the pelvis, was more or less answered by the operation of internal podalic version, or 'the handy operation'. What to do about cephalic presentations when there was obstruction to a labour was much more difficult. Although podalic version could be tried it was obviously not always successful. It can, in fact, be impossible if the uterus is contracting strongly and the liquor amnii has drained away. In such a situation forcible attempts to turn the baby are liable to rupture the uterus. Until the 20th century that meant certain death of the mother.

The use of the lever was unsatisfactory since not enough purchase could be obtained on a head that was stuck in the pelvis. The same applies to the vectis. This was similar to the later blade of the forceps but was much curved at its end. Like the lever this was intended to be applied to the occiput or some other part of the head on which purchase could be obtained so that the head could be drawn or levered out of the birth canal. The crotchet or hook killed the baby if it was not already dead. There is not enough room in the pelvis for both hands at the same time, so they could not be used to effect delivery. One hand alone cannot obtain sufficient purchase on the head either.

The answer to the problem of difficult cephalic delivery came with the invention of the obstetric forceps. It was essentially the brainchild of perhaps several members of the Chamberlen (there are several different spellings) family. It was kept a secret by them for about 100 years.

Dr William Chamberlen of Paris was a Huguenot protestant who fled to England with his family after the massacre of St Bartholomew's Eve in 1572. Catholics had put to death 50,000 Protestants. Chamberlen settled in Southampton. He had a son, Peter I, who remained as a medical practitioner in Southampton until his father died c.1596. He then went to London to join his younger brother, Peter II. Both became members of the Barber-Surgeons Company by passing an oral examination and paying fees. They were later upbraided by the Company for not attending lectures. They fell foul of the Royal College of Physicians too. It was the physicians who felt they had the right to control all forms of medical practice in London, looking on other practitioners as their ancillaries. Peter II was threatened with imprisonment by them because he had altered a prescription of a Dr Argent.

Peter II's son, Peter III, went to Cambridge and Padua to gain an MD degree which was a requirement to become a Fellow of the Royal College of Physicians. This honour was conferred on him in 1628, by which time his father had died, though his uncle, Peter I, was still alive. He was then aged about 70 and was called to attend Queen Henrietta Maria when she miscarried at Greenwich. He introduced Peter III to Court and it was he who probably attended at the birth of Charles II in 1630.

It was Peter III who suggested to the Royal College in 1634 that they should set up a body to instruct and regulate midwives. They turned the idea down and on hearing that he practised midwifery they averred that the subject was 'more properly the work of a surgeon'. They had heard, too, that in conducting his midwifery practice he used 'instruments of iron'. These were probably an early version of the obstetric forceps.

After a time in the Netherlands and because of failure to attend meetings of the Royal College Peter III was deprived of his Fellowship. He retired to Woodham Mortimer Hall, near Maldon in Essex. He probably practised midwifery there. Prudently he remained in the country during the time of the Commonwealth under Oliver Cromwell. He had been associated with the Court of Charles I who had been beheaded in Whitehall in 1649.

It was in an attic of Woodham Mortimer Hall that Peter III's forceps were found in 1813, hidden under floorboards. They had probably been put there by his widow, when he died in 1683. He had attempted to get back into the service of the Court at the restoration of the monarchy in 1660. There was delay about this but he managed to get his son Hugh appointed as physician in ordinary to the king in 1673. Hugh was one of 14 sons and four daughters of Peter III. He knew of and used the forceps. He had obtained a licence to practise midwifery in London from the bishop. In 1670 he went to Paris to demonstrate the use of the forceps to François Mauriceau. He boasted that he could deliver any woman with his instrument, but Mauriceau had given him a tiny rachitic dwarf to operate on and he failed to deliver her. However the secret was not revealed since the procedure was conducted under the cover of clothes and cloths.

On returning to London, Hugh translated Mauriceau's book on midwifery in 1673. He gained considerable financial advantage from it, but that was in his scheming nature. In the 17th chapter Hugh added his own commentary after condemning the use of the crotchet and the hook,

> 'But I can neither approve of that practice or these delays, because my father, brothers and myself (though none else in Europe as I know) have, by God's blessing and our own industry, attained to and long practised a way to deliver women in this case without any prejudice to them or their infants; though all others (being obliged for want of such an expedient to use the common way) do and must endanger, if not destroy, one or both with hooks. By this manual operation a labour may be dispatched (on the least difficulty) with fewer pains and sooner to the great advantage, and without danger, both of the woman and child'. (Walter Radcliffe, *The Secret Instrument*, Heinemann p.25.)

However, he would not explain anything further about the instrument, for it was a secret of his father, brothers and himself, so it was not 'my own to dispose of, nor publish it without injury to them'. This was the first published mention of the forceps. It may now seem reprehensible to have kept such a secret to themselves but in those days it was usual to maintain silence about one's own potions, nostrums and procedures, in order to attract practice and make money.

Hugh was held in some esteem for he became a Fellow of the Royal Society where he was a contemporary of Newton, Pepys and Sir Christopher Wren. In the records of the Society he is described as holding an MD. He was accoucheur to James II's queen, Mary, when she went into premature labour in June 1688 at Greenwich. He failed to get to her in time for the delivery and this led to the rumour that a baby had been smuggled into the bedchamber by the midwife in a warming-pan. There seems, however, to be no truth in this. It would have been almost impossible to achieve in a crowded room where so many were present as witnesses.

In November of 1688 James II was deposed, and William of Orange and Mary, (elder daughter of James) were invited to the throne. She had no children but her younger sister, later Queen Anne, who had a disastrous obstetric history of 15 pregnancies but produced no heir or heiress, was attended by Hugh.

Hugh proceeded on knavish and hypocritical ways and proposed a land bank, a national health service and the union of Scotland with England. He hoped to profit from all these but the land bank scheme was thought to be fraudulent and he had to flee the country to settle in Amsterdam in 1699. A jingle of the time about Hugh ran,

> 'To give you his character truly complete,
> He's doctor, projector, man-midwife and cheat.'

Hugh had a son, Hugh II (1664–1728), who acquired an MD degree and became a Fellow of the Royal College of Physicians. It was in his lifetime that the forceps became more widely known and used by other doctors. It was not directly through Hugh II that this happened but through three doctors from Essex where Peter III had lived and probably worked. These three were Edmund Chapman, William Giffard and Benjamin Pugh. None was further than 25 miles from Woodham Mortimer, the Chamberlen home.

Edmund Chapman produced his book *Essay for the Improvement of Midwifery. Chiefly with regard to the operation, to which are added 50 cases selected from upwards of 25 years' practice in 1733 from Red Lion Square*. He had by then moved to London from South Halstead. There was a description of the forceps in the book but no depiction of them. He was criticised for this, so in the edition of 1735 there is an excellent drawing of them. He gave their dimensions,

> 'Their length in a Right Line, Fifteen inches. The length of the Bows from the Joint, where the two parts cross, to the Upper Extremity, in a Right Line, Nine Inches and one Quarter. The Girt of the Bows, when shut, is, in the widest Part, Eight Inches.'

These are roughly the dimensions of the modern forceps. Moreover the picture shows the blades as being fenestrated, partly for lightness and partly in order to obtain a better grip on the fetal head. Previous attempts at making forceps had often had the blades solid. Another interesting point is that the blades already had a pelvic curve, adapted to the shape of the birth canal, as well as a cephalic one to hold the head.

Such a pelvic curve is frequently attributed to André Levret (1703–1780) of France at a later date. This may, in fact, have been an innovation made by Chapman, for the Chamberlen forceps found at Woodham Mortimer were straight-bladed.

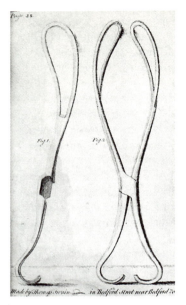

Fig. 6.1: Chapman's Forceps.

Another important feature of the instrument was that the lock where the shanks of each half cross over could be dismantled. Previous attempts such as that of Jean Palfyn (1650–1730) of Ghent in Belgium with his *mains de fer* had had parallel handles, shanks and blades, but there was no good way to hold them together to get a grip on the head. Yet other attempts had made the lock fixed by a screw as in a pair of scissors. But this will not do because the blades have to be opened so wide that they cannot be got into the pelvis except with great difficulty. The brilliance of the forceps as described by Chapman is that each half of the instrument is inserted into the pelvis separately, sliding to each side of the head in turn, and then they were, and are, only locked together after each was in place. However an unusual feature of the way in which he inserted the blades was that the first was inserted under the symphysis pubis and the second in the hollow of the sacrum. It may be that he was especially familiar with what became known as 'deep transverse arrest' of the head, when the occiput is lateral.

In Chapman's time the lock was held firmly by a removable pin, just as in a pair of scissors. But on one occasion Chapman lost the pin among all the clothes and he found that the forceps worked rather better without the pin than with it. He said,

> 'I do ingenuously confess, that I came by this Hint and Improvement by mere Accident, as, I believe, is frequently the Case in Discoveries of the greatest Importance. For many years my Forceps happen'd to be made of so soft a Metal as to bend and give way, or suffer some Alteration in their Curve. They were made, as usual, with the Screw fixed to one Part or Side of them. These I used

for some Years; but they often happening to slip off sideways (as before mentioned) my Opinion of the Instrument was so much lessened, that for many Years after I used it but seldom, and even not once in the Space of Ten Years. During which Time, when the Child could not be turned, I employed the Fillet only. This I freely communicated to a very ingenious Practitioner, now living in the Country, who will, I doubt not, readily remember on reading this. At length I caused another Pair to be made me, of better Metal, and some other Improvements; the Screw Part being contrived to take out, and not fixed, as in the former. This Screw I happened to lose in the cloths at the Delivery of a Woman, who, with her Child, is now living in Health in Town; and being sent for to another presently after, and being indeed forced to make the Trial, found that the Instrument did its office much better without the Screw, or the two Parts being fixt. All I can say in Praise of this noble Instrument, must necessarily fall short of what it justly demands. Those only, who have used it, and experienced the Excellency of it to their own Advantage, and the Security of their Offspring, can be truly sensible of its real Worth. As I think my self in Duty bound to recommend it strongly to the Gentlemen of my Profession, I shall omit no Opportunity of endeavouring to do it Justice.'

How right he was. The forceps used worldwide must now have saved the lives of hundreds of thousands, probably millions, of women and their babies. It might justly be claimed that it is among the most beneficent instruments ever devised for use in medicine. These were, of course, pre-anaesthetic days, but forceps, with gentleness, can be used without the woman being aware of them, when the head is low in the pelvis. Chapman was probably able to do this often. Moreover he used them too for the after-coming head in breech delivery, sometimes after performing internal podalic version.

When the baby was certainly dead Chapman was prepared to use the hook. In fact the handles of his forceps were recurved to form a hook, to be used when delivery otherwise failed. He wrote cautiously,

'I would of all things advise the *Operator* to be particularly cautious in his Enquiry whether the Infant in the Womb be *dead* or not; if he chuses to employ the *hook*, or the Child does not lie low enough for the Use of the *Forceps*, and the Parts are so straightened, that he cannot easily turn it; for there have been many deplorable Instances of Infants that have been drawn out this way as *dead*, whilst they have been really *living*. *Deventer* himself tells us, that he delivered a Woman, as he thought, of a *dead* Child, when to his great Surprize, and beyond his Expectation, the miserable Infant, who had been but roughly used, filled his ears with its *Cries* and *lamentations*. Some infants as Dr *Chamberlen* observes, have been drawn forth alive, after they have been thought to be dead, with both *Arms*, or some other Limb lopped off; and others miserably killed with the Use of *Crotchets* who might have been born alive, if no Mistake had been committed. A Man therefore should use his utmost Endeavour not to be deceived always remembring, with the above-mentioned Author, "That *Timidity* is, in this Case, more pardonable than *Temerity*: and that it is better to be deceived in treating a *dead* Infant as if it were *alive*, than a living one as if it were *dead*."'

The practice of midwifery must often have been horrifying in those days. Chapman discusses many other aspects of labour and delivery. He knew of spurious labour and advised performing vaginal examinations to make sure that the cervix was dilating. He mentioned the cord being round the neck and recommended that it might be cut and the ends held in the fingers until a ligature could be applied. He knew of the circulation of the blood in the baby and thought there must be some communication of the vessels of the mother with those of her fetus. For antepartum haemorrhage he knew that the only treatment was to empty the uterus as soon as possible. Because of this he performed manual removal of the placenta after delivery of the baby in every case. This was a common practice of the time. Most often he found that the placenta had separated and was lying in the cervix or at the top of the vagina.

In breech delivery he used groin traction with a finger when the legs were extended. In this he was a pioneer, since most others always tried to bring down the feet. He always brought down both extended arms, which was not the practice of many others. He delivered the head by putting a finger in the mouth to flex it, at the same time as drawing on the shoulders with his fingers. In twins he always extracted the second baby by the feet without waiting.

Chapman was a most remarkable man-midwife, and he exemplifies much of the best practice of the first half of the 18th century. He ends his book,

> 'But before I take my Leave of this Subject, if my *junior* Brethren, and the Gentlewomen in the Practice of *Midwifery*, will excuse me the Freedom, I would advise, and endeavour to influence them to behave both in *Words* and *Action*, with all imaginable Tenderness to such as fall under their Care. Their Pains both in *Mind* and *Body*, are at that time very hard upon them, and their Condition calls for the softest Manner in the necessary Assistance; especially where a Child requires *Alteration of Posture*, &c. And this as well with the *Poor* as others.'

William Giffard (d. 1731) was in similar mould to Chapman, who mentions him. He described his first time of using the forceps as being on 6th April 1726. This may or may not be earlier than Chapman, though Chapman's first case seems to have been in 1723. Giffard's book was *Cases in Midwifery written by the late Mr William Giffard, surgeon and man-midwife. Revised and published by Edward Hody MD, and Fellow of the Royal Society*. It appeared in 1734. Claims of priority for Chapman or Giffard are unnecessary. They knew each other and indeed Chapman wrote of his picture of the forceps that it was 'very little different from that used by the late Mr William Giffard'.

Benjamin Pugh is of interest because he, too, came from Essex, close to where Peter Chamberlen III worked. His book was entitled *A Treatise of Midwifery, chiefly with regard to the operation with several improvements in that art. To which is added some cases and descriptions of several new instruments both in Midwifery and Surgery*, by Benjamin Pugh, surgeon at Chelmsford in Essex, London, 1754. This was 21 years after Chapman's first edition.

It is fascinating now to contemplate that this marvellous instrument was kept secret for about 100 years, and then knowledge of it only slowly seeped out by a process of diffusion from rural Essex. Over the years the forceps have transformed the practice of midwifery. It was at about this time that there came to be increasing interest in the configuration of the bones of the pelvis. Arantius (1530–1589) had discussed smallness of the pelvis and other deformities in 1564. But the first major investigation of this branch of anatomy came from Hendrik van Deventer (1651–1724) of Amsterdam and The Hague. In 1701 he published *Operationes Chirurgicae Novum Lumen Exhibentes Obstetricantibus* (Surgical operations throwing new light on obstetrics). It was translated into English in 1716 when it became 'The Art of Midwifery Improved'. But it was often referred to as 'New Light for Midwives', showing their importance as against that of doctors in the management of childbirth. This suggests that the battles which marred relationships between midwives and doctors had begun even then.

Deventer described the pelvis more or less as we know it now. He was unsure whether the pubic bones separated during labour. But oddly he was sure that the coccyx and the sacrum swung rearwards and he therefore recommended that both bones should be pressed back manually to assist labour. He also persisted in thinking that the baby forced its own way out of the birth canal. So he had no idea of the importance of uterine contractions, nor of the actions of the abdominal muscles in the second stage of labour.

Deventer did describe the plane of the inlet, the pelvic cavity as an irregular cylinder, and the outlet in two planes at an angle based on the ischial tuberosities. The descriptions have lasted till the present day. He described contraction at the brim and also general contraction throughout the pelvis.

John Maubray (d. 1732) of London in 1724 produced a book with a very long-winded title which was fortunately abbreviated to *The Female Physician*. In it he suggested that midwives should have an understanding of the types of pelvis, and he recognized deep, large, broad, flat, oval and round shapes of the pelvic brim. He did not, however, relate these to any difficulties in labour. He attributed monsters (any abnormal baby) to indecent conjugal relations. He affected to see a monster run all over the deck of a ferry on the Zuyder Zee, and called it a 'moodiwarp'.

Maubray made a plea for Lying-in Hospitals.

> "Tis true we have hospitals for all other sorts of indigent people, and those indeed most superb and magnificent, and in every respect superior to others: only on this point of provision for poor miserable women in the time of their natural affliction, when they are in no case in a condition to help themselves, we have been hitherto and are still deficient, notwithstanding the excellent good precedents set before our eyes in foreign countries'.

He undertook a series of lectures on midwifery twice a week from his home in New Bond Street. He tried to arrange for his pupils to obtain experience 'in the touch' by which he meant vaginal examinations.

Sir Richard Manningham (1690–1759), also of London, mainly practising in Jermyn Street, established the first lying-in beds in England in a house next to his own. With many changes over time these became the basis of Queen Charlotte's Hospital. In 1720 he became a Licentiate of the Royal College of Physicians, so, at least for him, they seem to have dropped their objections to physicians conducting a midwifery practice. In 1739 he published his *Compendium Artis Obstetricariae* (Compendium of the Art of Obstetrics). It was later translated into English. Like Deventer he scouted the idea that obliquity of the uterus was a cause of difficult labour. At that time there were probably many women who had borne several babies and had very lax abdominal walls, allowing the pregnant uterus much mobility. He supported Deventer in recommending that the sacrum and coccyx should be pushed back in labour. He was much for internal podalic version when the head was stuck in the pelvis. It would seem that he knew little of the progress being made with the forceps at the time. He said that caesarean section was invariably fatal.

Both Manningham and Maubray discussed the chances of survival of babies born in the seventh and eighth months of pregnancy. Those born at seven months were under a lucky number according to astrologers. Those born in the eighth month were weak and sickly and unlikely to live. If they did they might be half-witted.

CHAPTER SEVEN

Eighteenth Century: William Smellie

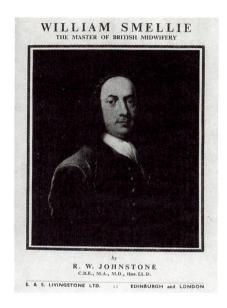

Fig. 7.1: Title page of 'William Smellie'

The towering figure in midwifery of the 18th century was William Smellie, a Scotsman who spent most of his working life in London. He became rightly known as the Master of British Midwifery. His classic work, which came out in 1752 was *A Treatise on the Theory and Practice of Midwifery.* Prior to this in 1742 was *A Course of Lectures upon Midwifery*, which was written to help his many students. Neither of these works contained illustrations. These were supplied in 1754 by his *Set of Anatomical Tables.*

He almost certainly knew of his contemporary in Dublin, Fielding Ould (1710–1789). He settled there after a spell in Paris under the tutelage of Grégoire. He obtained a Licence in Midwifery from the College of Physicians in Dublin. Although they conducted examinations for students of medicine at Trinity College they refused to examine Ould because he practised midwifery. However Trinity awarded him an MD in 1761, whereupon the Physicians wrote to the College saying that, 'as your College has thought proper to grant a degree in our Faculty to a person who had no academic education, and whom you know to be disqualified by his occupation for a licence to practice in our profession' they would in future withdraw their cooperation. By the time of the award of the MD, Ould had been Master of the Rotunda Hospital, perhaps the most prestigious obstetric post in Ireland and recognized internationally. The bigotry of the physicians of this time all over the British Isles is now beyond comprehension.

A

TREATISE

ON THE

Theory and Practice

OF

MIDWIFERY.

By W. SMELLIE, M.D.

LONDON:

Printed for D. Wilson, at Plato's Head, near
Round-Court, in the Strand.
MDCCLII.

*Fig. 7.2: Title page of William Smellie's
'A Treatise on the Theory and Practise
of Midwifery'*

But the Dublin College did grant Ould a Licence in Medicine in 1785 when he had been Master for 26 years. In that same year he was knighted by the Lord-Lieutenant of Ireland! A pleasing jingle of the time ran,

'Sir Fielding Ould is made a knight,
He should have been a lord by right;
For then each lady's prayer would be
"O, Lord, good Lord, deliver me."'

Whatever the Physicians thought there is little doubt that he was held in great esteem by ordinary Dubliners. In 1742, and only 32, Ould produced *A Treatise in Midwifery in Three Parts by Fielding Ould, Man-midwife*. A remarkable section of it was on the mechanism of labour, which describes the movements of the fetus as it is driven down the birth canal by the uterine contractions. In the most usual pelvis the long axis of the brim is a transverse oval, so the head fits into this diameter. As the head descends into the cavity the occiput moves to the front so that that part of the skull emerges under the symphysis pubis, in conformity with the pelvic outlet which has its longest diameter from front to back. The shoulders undergo similar rotation, after engaging in the brim transversely, so that at the outlet a shoulder also emerges from under the symphysis. As the shoulders rotate so does the head outside the vulva, thus keeping the axes of the shoulders and head at a right angle to one another. The understanding of the mechanism of labour means that if assistance of the birth is required it may be designed to mimic, as far as possible, the natural mechanisms.

Ould dismissed the idea that obliquity of the uterus had anything to do with difficult labour, and he disagreed with Deventer that the sacrum swung backwards during delivery, but he advocated pressing the coccyx back out of the way of the descending head. He delivered the second of twins immediately, after performing internal version if necessary. He delivered the placenta by pulling gently on the cord. After ten minutes, if this failed, he performed manual removal.

He used the forceps which he said in 1742, 'is in general use all over Europe'. This is only nine years after Chapman's description so the good news had travelled fast, far and wide. It was he who introduced episiotomy, in which when the perineal muscles are holding up delivery of the head they are incised with scalpel or scissors, away from the anus to prevent tearing into that part and the rectum. Repair of such a wound often failed in those days but that was better than having a tear extend into the rectum which could leave the woman incontinent of faeces thereafter.

Ould regarded caesarean section as, 'a detestable, barbarous, illegal piece of inhumanity', but he recognized that it might have to be done when there was a small contracted pelvis. He did this realizing that the operation might save the child but be mortal for the mother. He asked that 'divines' should give moral guidance in such cases. Midwifery has many moral aspects on which conflicting views are held and this was an early attempt to face them.

William Smellie (1695–1763) went to London in 1738 from his practice in Lanark, just south of both Edinburgh and Glasgow, because he had heard of the use of the forceps as described by Chapman. He had tried out the instrument in 1737 and found it unsatisfactory. He was not very satisfied with what he discovered in London either, saying, 'here I saw nothing was to be learned'. This may seem a harsh judgement but he was already very experienced. He then went to Paris to see the younger Grégoire, who had a high reputation, but Smellie was disappointed in his quest there too. But he did learn something of the use of models for teaching purposes. The exact nature of these is not known.

By 1741 Smellie was in London and began teaching. His advertisement in the *London Evening Post* of 1st June that year read,

> 'On Monday, 14th. June, at 5 pm, will begin a course of lectures on the theory and practice of Midwifery, at 11 am for women, and 3 pm for men, by Mr Smellie, at his house in the New Court, formerly the Key and Garter Tavern, over against St Albans Street, Pall Mall.'

He later moved his practice to Leicester Square. It is especially to be noted that he intended to teach both men and women. Over the years he records that he had 900 students 'exclusive of female students'.

The Treatise arose out of these lectures. They were supplemented by,

> 'reference to the working of those machines which I have contrived to resemble and represent real women and children; and on which all kinds of different labours are demonstrated, and even performed by every individual student'.

Perhaps his 'machines' in some way resembled the bony pelves and mannikins which every midwifery student now uses as educational and training aids.

The Treatise was differently arranged from the Lectures because these had been illustrated by the models, whereas the Treatise had no illustrations. He wrote, 'I have ... industriously avoided all theory, except so much as may serve to whet the genius of young practitioners, and be as hints to introduce more valuable discoveries in the art.' In his series of courses 1,150 poor women were attended 'by the stated collection of my pupils: over and above those to which we were often called by midwives, for the relief of the indigent.'

Smellie justified himself on the basis of this extensive experience which 'will, I hope, screen me from the imputation of arrogance, with regard to the task I have undertaken'. The introduction expertly reviews all previous literature. He spoke well of Paré, Mauriceau, Lamotte, Chapman, Giffard, Ould and many others. There are four books within the Treatise. The first dealt with the bones of the pelvis. He gave the measurements of the brim, cavity and outlet. They are essentially those accepted today. He drew special attention to the shape of the brim and the outlet, the first having the major diameter transverse, and the second from before backwards. On abnormal pelves he attributes the majority to rickets, describing the rachitic pelvis very exactly. He described the features of the fetal head which can be felt on vaginal examination. From these he described the normal mechanism of labour.

The anatomy of the soft parts of the pelvis are well described, including the broad ligaments and peritoneum as well as the vessels of the uterus. He quoted the results of injections of them. He noted that the musculature of the uterus does not get thinner in pregnancy as others had often believed.

Smellie had difficulty, which he acknowledged in understanding menstruation and conception. But he believed that an ovum was discharged from the ovary and was conveyed along the Fallopian tube, 'by a vermicular [worm-like] or peristaltic motion; and if it is not immediately impregnated with an *Animalcule* of the male semen, must be dissolved and lost ...'. The animalcules he referred to were the spermatozoa which had been seen under the microscope by Leeuwenhoek. But he knew he did not know much for he wrote,

> 'notwithstanding the plausibility of the scheme, it is attended with circumstances which are hitherto inexplicable; namely the manner in which the *Animalculum* gains admission into the *Ovum*, either while it remains in the *Ovarium*, sojourns in the tube, or is deposited in the *Fundus Uteri* ...'.

Smellie could not explain the onset of labour either. He made a stab at it but was aware that his explanation was not a very good one, but,

> 'it nevertheless seems more probable than that hypothesis, which imputes labour pains, to the motion of the child calcitrating [kicking] the *Uterus*: for, it frequently happens, that the woman never feels the child stir during the whole time of labour, and dead children are delivered as easily as those that come alive ...'.

This is a most telling observation and totally destructive of the ancient theory. He scouted the notion that babies born at the seventh or eighth month of gestation were stronger than those born at the ninth month. 'Experience, however, contradicts this assertion; for the older the child is, we find it always (*caeteris paribus*) the stronger, consequently the more hardy and easily nursed ...'. There was an old notion that the placenta was always attached to the fundus of the uterus, but he had found it attached to all parts on different occasions.

Book II deals with diseases of pregnant women. He treated nausea by bleeding, which shows that he subscribed to notions of plethora, an old idea which attributed many illnesses to an excess of blood. He even went so far as to bleed women suffering from antepartum haemorrhage, which could only have compounded the problem of severe blood loss. He removed 8–12 ounces of blood. On the other hand he knew that the only way to stem the bleeding was to have the uterus empty of all its contents. In these cases he said, 'but above all things opiates must be administered, to procure rest, and quiet the uneasy apprehensions of the mind ...'. Of convulsions he says remarkably little, except to say they should be treated by bleeding and blisters, both of them ancient remedies.

Book III discusses the position of the fetus within the womb. It is, of course, that of the general flexion of the body, with the chin on the chest. He said that the usual position was for the baby to have its head presenting over the brim for almost the whole of pregnancy. Many other authors believed that it was more usual for the head to be in the fundus for most of the pregnancy, turning to cephalic later.

The chapters on labour distinguish between true and false labour especially by observing the progressive dilatation of the cervix by 'touching', i.e. vaginal examination, using one finger only, not two. Two fingers always cause the woman to complain he said. He divided labours into natural, non-natural and praeternatural. The meaning of natural births is obvious enough,

> 'in which the head presents and the woman is delivered without extraordinary help; those births are called laborious or nonnatural, when the head comes along with difficulty, and must be assisted either with the hand in opening the parts, or with the fillet or forceps, or even where there is a necessity for opening [the head] and extracting with the crotchet; and those in which the child is brought by the breech or feet, are denominated praeternatural [out of the ordinary course of nature] because the delivery is performed in a praeternatural way.'

This is an easy enough classification to understand. It corresponds to the normal births, malpresentations of the head, and breech and transverse presentations of today.

Smellie knew the significance of each form of birth,

> 'As the head, therefore, presents right in nine hundred and twenty of a thousand labours, all such are to be accounted natural; those of the other seventy, that require assistance may be deemed laborious; and the other ten, to be denominated laborious or praeternatural, as they are delivered by the head or feet.'

He discussed the various positions a woman might take up during labour. 'The *London* method is very convenient in natural and easy labours; the patient lies in bed upon one side, the knees being contracted to the belly, and a pillow put between them to keep them asunder.' But later there is the kind advice, 'She is commonly laid upon the left side, but in this particular she is to consult her own ease …'. He suggested the possibilities of the *Parisian* method with the woman half sitting and half lying but he thought that sometimes other positions, 'such as standing or kneeling, ought to be tried …'. 'Nevertheless, the patient must by no means be too much fatigued.' However, 'in the description of all laborious and praeternatural deliveries treated of in this performance, the reader must suppose the woman lying on her back …'.

Smellie was conservative in preserving the fore-waters as long as possible, and he noted that when they broke it was easier to feel the sutures and fontanelles on the fetal head. When the cervix would not dilate he advocated slow and gradual stretching of it with the whole hand in the vagina. 'This dilatation, however, ought to be cautiously performed, and never attempted except when absolutely necessary; even then it must be effected slowly, and in time of a pain, when the woman is least sensible of the dilating force.'

After delivery he thought that if the baby cried soon the cord should be cut, but if breathing should be slow in starting, 'the operation of tying and cutting must be delayed …'. If as a result of moulding of the skull bones the baby had convulsions he recommended once again that there should be bleeding to the extent of two or three large spoonfuls.

For delivering the placenta Smellie thought that the maternal end of the cord should not be tied so that blood could drain away, thus reducing the size of the placenta. It was then to be withdrawn by gently pulling on the cord. Failing that, the hand was to be inserted in the vagina and usually the placenta would be found there or in the lower part of the cervix. If not, he advocated that manual removal of the placenta from the uterine wall should be done, squeezing the hand up into the form of a cone to get it through the cervix or through a rare hour-glass constriction. He knew that the afterbirth could be left inside for several days but then, 'if the Uterus should be inflamed from any accident, and the woman be lost, the operator will be blamed for leaving the after-birth behind.'

After normal labours, Smellie proceeded to discuss *laborious labours* and the use of the forceps.

> 'A general outcry hath been raised against gentlemen of the profession, as if they delighted in using instruments and violent methods in the course of their practice; and this clamour hath proceeded from ignorance of such as do not know that instruments are sometimes absolutely necessary, or from the interested views of some low, obscure and illiterate practitioners, both male and female, who think they find their account in decrying the practice of their neighbours. It is not to be denied, that mischief has been done by instruments in the hands of the unskilful and unwary, but I am persuaded, that every judicious practitioner will do everything for the safety of his patients before he has recourse to any violent method, either with the hand or instrument; though cases will occur, in which gentle methods will absolutely fail. It is therefore necessary to explain

these reinforcements which must be used in dangerous labours; though they ought by no means to be called in, except when the life of the mother or child, or both, is evidently at stake; and even then managed with the utmost caution; for my own part, I have always avoided them as far as I thought consistent with the safety of my patients, and strongly inculcated the same maxim upon those who have submitted to my instructions.'

He outlined the causes of difficult labour as great weakness due to vomiting, diarrhoea, floodings or other diseases; excessive grief or anxiety; rigidity of the cervix or vagina; a small distorted pelvis; hardness of the head or hydrocephalus; wrong presentation; and constriction of the uterus in front of the head.

If the head was just above the brim he recommended that internal podalic version should be performed. If the head is 'pressed into the middle or lower part of the *Pelvis*, and the *Uterus* strongly contracting, delivery ought to be performed with the forceps ... we must determine when we ought to wait patiently for the efforts of nature, and when it is absolutely necessary to come to her aid.'

There has always been the problem of the baby's versus the mother's interests. 'Doubtless it is our duty to save both mother and child, if possible; but if that is impracticable, to pay our chief regard to the parent: and in all dubious cases, to act cautiously and circumspectly, to the best of our judgment and skill.' He criticised the way in which previous operators simply applied the blades of the forceps to any part of the head, whereas he 'began to consider the whole in a mechanical view, and reduce the extraction of the child to the rules of moving bodies in different direction ...'. Here he emphasized the importance of the mechanism of labour as Ould had done. Smellie applied the blades over the ears and in conformity with the long axis of the head.

With the head above the brim he did try the fillet or bandage. This was a system of loops which were supposed to slip over the head, under the chin and occiput, but he found it difficult to apply as all other operators have done. Because he wished to discourage his pupils and himself from trying to apply forceps to the high head, which is dangerous, 'I have always used and recommended the forceps so short in the handles, that they cannot be used with such violence as will endanger the woman's life ...'.

Smellie's most famous contribution was to define the rules for applying the forceps. The head was to be low down. The cervix was to be fully dilated, made to be so by manual dilatation if need be. The position of the head in the pelvis was to be known by feeling the sutures and fontanelles and preferably an ear. The forceps should be applied along the ears if at all possible.

The application of the forceps was to take place under the cover of a sheet. He kept each half of the instrument in separate pockets of his coat. 'At any rate, as women are commonly frightened at the very name of an instrument, it is advisable to conceal them as much as possible, until the character of the operator is fully established.' He said, 'by which means he will often be able to deliver with the forceps, without their being perceived by the woman herself, or any other of the assistants'. This is true. To prevent the metallic sound of the forceps he had them wrapped in leather strips.

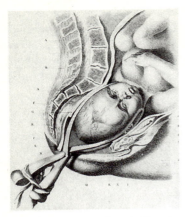

Figure 7.3: From 'Obstetric Plates' by William Smellie

With the forceps applied he pulled on them, after lashing the handles together, only with each uterine contraction. To help the baby negotiate the curve of the birth canal he stood up to draw the head out and upwards. He always tried to mimic the natural mechanism of labour even when that meant rotating the head within the pelvic cavity.

For face presentations he thought the best procedure was to perform internal podalic version. If that failed and there was no progress he had to resort to the crotchet. He listed the signs of intrauterine fetal death as the fetus not moving; the passage of meconium; no pulsation in the fontanelles or temporal artery; swelling on the scalp (caput succedaneum); laxity of the skull bones; foetid secretions from the vagina; no movement of the tongue when a finger is placed in the mouth; no pulsations in the cord; and several others. Not all are diagnostic. Some are not in fact signs of fetal death. Praeternatural labours were essentially a matter of conducting breech delivery. He tended to bring down the legs, but in extended breech he used groin traction. Normally he did not bring down the arms unless there was delay. By rotating the body after its delivery he brought the occiput to the front. Then he used jaw flexion and shoulder traction to bring out the head. All these manoeuvres had, of course, been described by earlier authors.

Smellie knew how difficult internal version could be for the operator.

'In all cases where the accoucheur foresees that great force will be requisite, he ought to save his strength as much as possible, beginning slowly, and resting his hand between whiles, during the operation of pushing up and turning the child in the *Uterus*: for, if he begins work in an hurry, and exerts his utmost strength at first, his hands will be so cramped and enervated, that he will be obliged to desist, and give them some respite; so that it may be a long time before he recovers the use of them, and even then they will be so much weakened as to be scarce able to effect delivery, which is thus impeded and delayed.'

Anyone who has performed intrauterine manipulations, even under anaesthesia, can vouch for the truth of this. For transverse lie he recommended internal version if that were

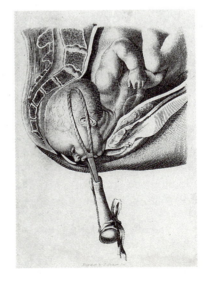

Figure 7.4: From 'Obstetric Plates' by William Smellie

possible, but if an arm or the cord had prolapsed and the baby was dead then decapitation was the only recourse. With twins he delivered the second one immediately after the first. Caesarean section sometimes had to be done when there were no other alternatives,

> 'in such emergencies, if the woman is strong, and of a good habit of body, the *Caesarian operation* is certainly adviseable, and ought to be performed; because the mother and child have no other chance to be saved, and it is better to have recourse to an operation which hath sometimes succeeded, than to leave them both to inevitable death. Nevertheless, if the woman is weak, exhausted with fruitless labour, violent floodings, or any other evacuation, which renders her recovery doubtful, even if she were delivered in the natural way: in these circumstances, it would be rashness and presumption to attempt an operation of this kind, which ought to be delayed until the woman expires, and then immediately performed, with a view to save the child.'

He describes the detail of the operation, of course of the classical variety through the upper segment, including the closure of the abdomen with sutures, though he does not mention repair of the uterine wall. It was uncommon then for this to be done.

For the lying-in period of one month he gives detailed instructions about the bed and its disposition as well as its coverings. The woman was not to have solid food for five or seven days but should be given

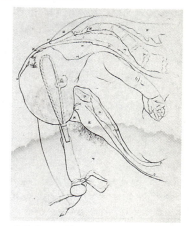

Figure 7.5: From 'Obstetric Plates' by William Smellie

> 'plentifully of warm, diluting fluids, such as barley-water, gruel, chicken-water and teas; caudles are also commonly used, composed of water-gruel boiled up with mace and cinnamon, to which, when strained, is added a third or fourth part of white wine ... sweetened with sugar to their taste ...'

Perspiration was to be encouraged, noise reduced to a minimum and anything which might cause 'dejection of spirits' was to be avoided.

Infection was called 'mortification' and if it were total 'the woman is soon destroyed'. Floodings in the puerperium were to be dealt with by removing pieces of placenta and encouraging the uterus to contract by warm cloths applied to the back and abdomen. Prolapse might have to be treated with a pessary. Vesico-vaginal fistula 'is an inexpressible inconvenience and misfortune to the poor woman, both from the smell and continual wetting of her cloaths'. His first approach was to keep the bladder empty with a catheter. He attempted repair with stitches after a time but it is unlikely that this would have been successful at that time.

The book closes on the theme of the qualifications of accoucheurs and midwives. The accoucheurs should be 'masters of anatomy, and acquire a competent knowledge in surgery and physick ...' and should learn obstetrics under a master,

> '... but over and above the advantages of education, he ought to be endued with a natural sagacity, resolution and prudence; together with that humanity which adorns the owner, and never fails of being agreeable to the distressed patient: in consequence of this virtue, he will assist the poor as well as the rich, behaving always with charity and compassion. He ought to act and speak with the utmost delicacy of decorum, and never violate the trust reposed in him, so as to harbour the least immoral or indecent design; but demean himself in all respects suitable to the dignity of his profession.'

'A Midwife, ... ought to be a decent, sensible woman, of a middle age, able to bear fatigue'. She needs to know of the bones of the pelvis 'with all the contained parts'. She must know how to 'touch' and of the various kinds of normal and abnormal labour.

> '... she ought to live in friendship with other women of the same profession, contending with them in nothing but in knowledge, sobriety, diligence, and patience; she ought to void all reflections upon men practitioners, and when she finds herself difficulted, candidly have recourse to their assistance: on the other hand, this confidence ought to be encouraged by the man, who, when called, instead of openly condemning her method of practice, (even though it should be erroneous) ought ... to rectify what is amiss, without exposing her mistakes. This conduct will as effectively conduce to the welfare of the patient, and operate as a silent rebuke upon the conviction of the midwife; who finding herself treated so tenderly, will be more apt to call for necessary assistance on future occasions, and to consider the accoucheur as a man of honour, and a real friend. These gentle methods will prevent that mutual calumny and abuse which too often prevail among the male and female practitioners, and redound to the advantage of both: for no accoucheur is so perfect, but that he may err sometimes; and on such occasions, he must expect to meet with retaliation from those midwives whom he may have roughly used.'

It is unfortunate that these words of his had to be written. The invention of the forceps and their wider use began to drive a wedge between accoucheurs and midwives. Their functions in the delivery rooms were complementary but came to be viewed as antagonistic. The advent of man-midwives with their instruments which were not used by midwives generated tension between them. Midwives, prior to this, had held the territory of the labour room as their own exclusive preserve and that was surely being encroached on, and so was resisted, often vehemently, and perhaps to the detriment of patients.

Elizabeth Nihell (b. 1723) was most incensed by Smellie. She was a famous midwife who practised from the Haymarket in London, not more than a few hundred yards from Leicester Square. No doubt Smellie took away some of the practice she considered to be hers. She had trained at the Hôtel Dieu in Paris and was married to a surgeon-apothecary. In 1760 she published *A Treatise on the Art of Midwifery, Setting Forth various Abuses therein, especially as to the Practice with Instruments, the whole serving to put all Rational Inquirers in a fair way of very safely forming their Own Judgment upon the Question which is it best to employ in Cases of Pregnancy and Lying-in, a Man-midwife or a Midwife.* Her invective knew few bounds. Smellie's pupils she referred to as 'broken barbers, tailors, or even pork butchers', '... and what are those arms by which they maintain themselves, but those instruments, those weapons of death!'

She called Smellie's known big hands 'the delicate fist of a great horse-godmother of a he-midwife'. She obviously saw and foresaw the power which the use of the forceps had put into the hands of the man-midwives. She attempted to ridicule everything that Smellie was and did, especially attacking the use of his teaching machines which she described as being made of wood with leather forming the abdominal wall, and with a bladder that represented the uterus.

It is sad that this tension between midwives and their male counterparts should have engendered such dissension. It was perhaps the start of the subject of obstetrics as distinct from that of midwifery. Both are still essential and are complementary to each other. Male and female helpers at childbirth have no need to be jealous of each other and their preserves.

CHAPTER EIGHT

Other Advances of the Eighteenth Century

Smellie perhaps best exemplifies the general state of the clinical art and practice of midwifery in the mid-18th century, because he dealt with the subject so comprehensively. There were many other observations and movements during the whole century which have had lasting effects on the development of midwifery.

There seems to have been a general social concern for the poor throughout the century. In 1741 the bluff sailor Thomas Coram started the Foundling Hospital in London, for sick children. The first lying-in beds in a general hospital were in the Middlesex Hospital in 1747. Prior to this the Rotunda Hospital in Dublin was built on the initiative of Bartholomew Mosse in 1745. William Shippen in Philadelphia opened a private maternity hospital in 1765. Edinburgh had a maternity hospital in 1784, founded by John Aitken. Many major general hospitals started in the first half of the 18th century too. The charitable impulse, evident at this time, may have gained christian impetus from the beginning of Methodism with John Wesley who began his ardent preaching around 1738. As regards lying-in hospitals the wider knowledge of the benefits of the obstetric forceps may have had an influence on where charity and concern for the poor might best be bestowed. An example of lying-in hospitals was the New Westminster Lying-in Hospital of John Leake's (1729–1792). It was built just across the newly erected Westminster Bridge in Lambeth, and opened its doors in 1767. It was essentially for the wives of soldiers and seamen who had been killed or wounded in the battles then being waged in the New World.

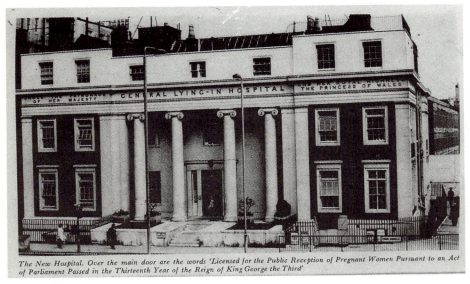

The New Hospital. Over the main door are the words 'Licensed for the Public Reception of Pregnant Women Pursuant to an Act of Parliament Passed in the Thirteenth Year of the Reign of King George the Third'

Fig. 8.1: The General Lying-in Hospital, York Road, Lambeth, London

Leake designed some strange forceps, but his especial interest seems to have been in training midwives and to a lesser extent doctors. His hospital became the General Lying-in Hospital, York Road, and it maintained its midwife training tradition for 200 years. Leake gave lectures and demonstrations, and issued certificates to those who completed the courses, which seems a very modern concept. There was practical work in labour for the students both within the hospital and in the homes of people in the surrounding district.

Admission to the care of the hospital either as in-patients or out-patients (cared for in their own homes) was by recommendation from one of the subscriber governors of the hospital. It was therefore not a matter of medical need but rather of obtaining charitable patronage. A pregnant woman had to petition a governor and obtain a certificate from him saying that she was a 'worthy object of the charity'.

A major problem for the hospital was the number of births to single women. They often absconded leaving their babies to be cared for by the hospital authorities. The usual recourse was to ask the Foundling Hospital to take them, but that was often full and overtaxed with work. The law required that babies born in a parish had to be looked after by that parish. The local councillors of Lambeth found this an increasing burden and complained bitterly to the governors of the Lying-in Hospital about it, but without much effect. However, it did lead for a time to the hospital refusing to admit unmarried mothers.

Infection in the puerperium was a serious worry for Leake and many others. It carried off a high percentage of women and those who did recover were often chronic invalids thereafter. There was, of course, no knowledge of bacteriology. Infection was deemed to be due to bad air. Leake therefore advocated good ventilation and he tried to prevent overcrowding in his wards. Those known to be infected were isolated when possible. Clothes and bedclothes were washed after an infected patient had used them, by in-house laundresses, who boiled linen in large copper vats in the basement. It was not uncommon then for the bedclothes not to be changed between succeeding occupants. Bartholomew Mosse of the Rotunda Hospital in Dublin pursued similar practices, cutting slots into window panes so that air had to circulate even with the windows shut, so outwitting patients and midwives.

Thomas Denman (1733–1815) of the Middlesex Hospital in 1765 published his *Essay on Puerperal Fever*, so there was general concern about the problem at that time. But Charles White (1728–1813) of Manchester was one who advanced practical knowledge of the subject. In 1773 came his, *A Treatise on the Management of Pregnant and Lying-in Women, and the Means of Curing, but more especially Preventing, the Principle Disorders to which they are Liable, together with some new directions concerning the delivery of the child and placenta in natural births.*

White insisted on free ventilation and movement of air in lying-in rooms. He wrote,

> 'When the woman is in labour, she is often attended by a number of her friends in a small room, with a large fire, which, together with her own pains, throw her into profuse sweats; by the heat of the chamber, and the breath of so many

people the whole air is rendered foul, and unfit for respiration; this is the case in all confined places, hospitals, jails and small houses, inhabited by many families, where fevers are apt to be generated, and proportionately the more so where there is the greatest want of air.'

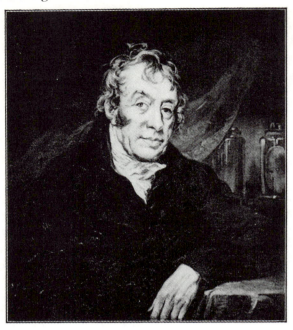

Fig. 8.2: Portrait of Charles White

This is a graphic description of the way in which labours were then conducted. It is interesting that he mentions hospitals and jails, in both of which infections frequently raged.

'As soon as she is delivered, if she be a person in affluent circumstances, she is covered up close in bed with additional clothes, the curtains are drawn round the bed, and pinned together, every crevice in the windows and door is stopped close, not excepting the keyhole, the windows are guarded not only with shutters and curtains, but even with blankets, the more effectively to exclude the fresh air, and the good woman is not suffered to put her arm, or even her nose out of bed, for fear of catching cold.'

For the poor, matters were even worse, for 'the dampness and closeness of their houses' and

> 'they are still in worse situation in hospitals, where a number are crowded, not only in one house, but in one ward, where the disease is conveyed from one to another by the putrid miasmata lodging in the curtains, bed clothes, and furniture, and by the necessary houses [earth closets], which are either contiguous to, or so near the hospital as to occasion a most disagreeable smell, and must of course convey that infection which cannot be more effectually communicated, than by excrements.'

This shows almost incredible prescience for one without knowledge of bacteria. He struggled with ideas of contagion and how infection might be carried by 'miasmata' from one person to another. There is also the surprising emphasis on excreta as vehicles of infection, though he was probably equating smell with the possibilities of infection, which is a notion still often found among those with no knowledge of bacteriology.

White recommended that few people should be in the labour room, which should be kept cool, screening the windows from the sun if need be. No fire should be lit except in the coldest weather. Windows and doors should be opened every day, and the baby should be kept in a separate room if possible. The baby should begin breastfeeding soon after birth. It was then not uncommon for babies not to be fed until four or five days after delivery. They too were stifled with far too many coverings in their cots. White also suggested that women should spend much of the day sitting up to aid the drainage of the lochia from the genital tract.

There is very clear evidence of the way in which his mind was working on the subject of infection in hospitals. He wrote,

> 'If separate apartments cannot be allowed to every patient, at least as soon as the fever has seized one she ought immediately to be moved into another room, not only for her immediate safety but that of other patients; or it would be still better if every woman were delivered in a separate ward and were to remain there a week or ten days until all danger of the fever is over ... Whenever a patient has recovered from this fever and is removed to another room, the bedding and curtains should be washed, the floor and woodwork cleansed with vinegar, and it would still add to the salubrity of the apartment if it were stoved with brimstone.'

In 1785 White gave a very good description of '*phlegmasia alba dolens*' – the painful white leg of the puerperium. It is probable that he did not understand that this was due to thrombosis of the deep veins, with accompanying constriction of the arteries which causes the whiteness.

White was a great surgeon and obstetrician. In 1752 he founded the Manchester Infirmary. After a quarrel with other governors he established in 1790 'a lying-in charity for attendance on poor married women in their own homes'. The emphasis on married women is to be noted. Unmarried pregnant women were objects of opprobrium everywhere. The charity later evolved into the renowned St. Mary's Hospital, Manchester. Such was his general fame that he was made a Fellow of the Royal Society in 1762.

The understanding of infection was taken a step further by Alexander Gordon (1752–1799) of Aberdeen. In 1795 he published *A Treatise on the Epidemic Puerperal Fever of Aberdeen*. He studied medicine in Edinburgh and Leyden and by 1781 he had become a member of the Company of Surgeons, after having served in the navy, rising to the rank of naval surgeon. In 1785 he retired on half pay and came under the tutelage of two doctors on the staff of the General Lying-in Hospital, York Road. He certainly became a friend of Thomas Denman (1733–1815) of the Middlesex Hospital, who had written about puerperal fever in 1768. Gordon's book was dedicated to Denman.

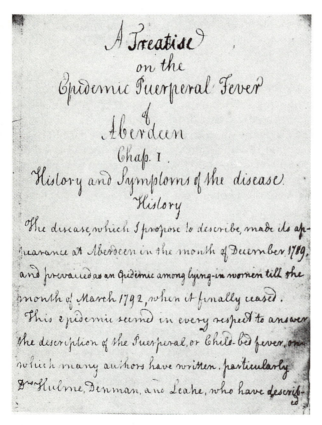

Fig 8.3: Manuscript beginning of 'A Treatise on the Epidemic Puerperal Fever of Aberdeen'

Gordon was awarded the MD of Aberdeen in 1788. Two years earlier he had been appointed to the Aberdeen Dispensary. This was a base for mainly out-patient practice where patients could come for treatment and were sometimes visited in their own homes. It was on the basis of his work there that Gordon came to his then startling conclusions.

An epidemic of puerperal fever raged in Aberdeen from December 1789 until March 1792. It affected women of all kinds, whatever their social status. Weather was not a determining factor.

> 'It prevailed principally among the lower classes of women and on account of my public office and extensive practice in midwifery, most of the cases came under my care. But women in the higher walks of life were not exempted, when they happened to be delivered by a midwife or physician who had previously attended any patients labouring under the disease ... by observation, I plainly perceived the channel by which it is propagated; and I arrived at that certainty in the matter, that I could venture to foretell what women would be affected with the disease, upon hearing by what midwife they were to be delivered or by what nurse they were to be attended during their lying-in; and almost in every instance my prediction was verified.'

He was able to do this because he kept a record of the names, ages and addresses of the patients and the names of those who attended them, both doctors and midwives, from December 1789 to October 1792. In the case of Mrs Jeffries and other country midwives he found that none of their cases developed the fever because they never tended anyone suffering from it.

Gordon noted that puerperal fever often occurred at the same time as the skin and wound inflammation of erysipelas, now known to be caused by streptococci. He knew that puerperal fever only occurred after birth because there was then a wound inside the uterus at the placental site.

He showed from his tables just who was carrying the disease from patient to patient and did not even exempt himself. 'It is a disagreeable declaration for me to mention that I myself was the means of carrying the infection to a great number of women.' Surprisingly he did not fully draw what now seem obvious conclusions about prevention. Rather he thought he had found a cure which consisted essentially of bleeding and purging. But he did advocate fumigation.

> 'The patient's apparel and bedclothes ought either to be burnt or thoroughly purified; and the nurses and physicians who have attended patients affected with puerperal fever, ought carefully to wash themselves and to get their apparel properly fumigated before it be put on again.'

The publication of his book did not endear Gordon to the midwives and doctors of Aberdeen. He was much reviled by them for showing them to be the carriers of infection. He described a case where his advice had been turned down and plaintively says, 'On this as well as on many other occasions I found that scientific practice and popular opinion very seldom correspond'.

Probably because of this clamour against him he returned to service in the Royal Navy in 1795, the year his Treatise was published. By August 1799 he had contracted tuberculosis, which was not uncommon in the overcrowded ships of the time. He died in December of that year at the age of 47.

In 1786 John Hunter, the famous surgeon, investigated venereal diseases. He inoculated himself with pus from a patient and now we know that from this he developed both syphilis and gonorrhoea, though he was not aware of the fact. However Benjamin Bell (1749–1806) of Virginia did differentiate these two diseases in his *Treatise on Gonorrhoea Virulenta and Lues Venerea* of 1793. This preliminary work became of importance later in obstetrics and gynaecology.

The forceps came into more general use after the mid-century. There was some opposition to them, sometimes from within the medical profession as well as by the midwives. One famous opponent, because of his literary connections, was Dr John Burton (1710–1771) of York. The year after Smellie's Treatise, 1753, Burton wrote *A Letter to William Smellie MD, Wherein the various Gross Mistakes and Methods of Practice mentioned and recommended by that Writer are fully demonstrated and generally corrected.* He objected to Fielding Ould's descriptions of the mechanism of labour too. Dr Burton is only remembered now because he is the character on which Dr Slop in Laurence Sterne's classic novel *Tristram Shandy* is modelled. He is there lampooned partly because he damaged Tristram's nose at birth with the forceps.

Other operations to deal with obstructed labour were devised. They were pubiotomy and symphysiotomy. The first operation was performed by sawing through one or both pubic bones (without anaesthesia of course) so that the two halves of the pelvis could be distracted by helpers to enlarge the diameters and so allow the head to go through. An alternative was to cut through the ligaments and cartilage of the symphysis with the same object in view. This last had a vogue for some time in Ireland. The forcible separation of the pelvic bones was inevitably hinged round the sacro-iliac joints, whose ligaments were permanently stretched. The result was backache thereafter and a waddling ungainly gait. Both barbarous operations, as well as caesarean section, even in that age, were roundly condemned by Denman, William Hunter, William Osborn and many others.

John Harvie (fl. 1767) succeeded William Smellie as a teacher at their house in Wardour Street. In 1767 he published *Practical Directions, shewing a method of preserving the perineum in birth and delivering the Placenta without violence.* The perineum was supported with a hand over a pad in the way almost universally accepted now. As regards the placenta he recognized that pulling on the cord could cause inversion of the uterus and that manual removal could cause collapse and shock. He called them both 'hurrying methods'. He advocated patience but had noticed that when the placenta had separated from its bed in the upper segment and moved downwards into the lower segment or vagina that the uterus became smaller, more mobile and rode up into the abdomen above the placenta. By pressing the uterus downwards the placenta would often be delivered, and the same manoeuvre could be used to expel clots. It is still often used. In some difficult cases he was, of course, prepared to use cord traction or even manual removal if delivery of the placenta had not been effected in about one hour. Small though this advance might now seem to be it greatly changed practice for the better, saving thousands of women from pain, shock and haemorrhage and subsequent infection caused by manual removal with its probable introduction of infection into the genital tract. It is remarkable too in that he examined the abdomen. This had been rarely done prior to this time. He noted that the presence of a second twin need not be diagnosed by vaginal examination, for 'by laying the hand upon the belly, a child, if there be one, is at once discovered'. It is astonishing now to realize how late abdominal examinations came on the midwifery scene.

Another pupil of Smellie's was William Hunter (1718–1783) who also followed him from Lanarkshire. He was especially interested in anatomy as well as midwifery. In 1741 he stayed with James Douglas, who in 1730 had described the peritoneal pouch named after him. Hunter became the most fashionable obstetrician of his day, and was appointed to the Middlesex Hospital for the 'care of the lying-in department'. Although an excellent man-midwife his main aim was to be 'a breeder of anatomists'. It was his success in this that brought his younger brother, John Hunter (1728–1793), to London. He became the founder of modern surgery in Britain, based to a great extent on anatomical researches. William Hunter published *The Anatomy of the Human Gravid Uterus* in 1774. It has a remarkable series of plates depicting dissections of the uterus and placenta with the fetus in situ. No previous work had done so in such detail.

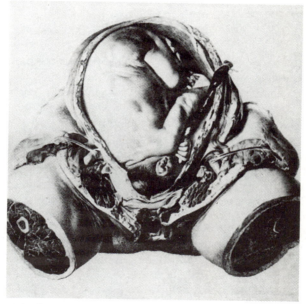

Fig. 8.4: 'The Anatomy of the Human Gravid Uterus' by William Hunter

Other scientific advances of indirect relevance to midwifery were a pathology classic of 1761 by Giovanni Battista Morgagni (1682–1771) of Padua, and another by Caspar Friedrich Wolff (1733–1794) of Berlin on embryology in 1759. Morgagni's work was *De Sedibus et Causis Morborum* (On the Sites and Causes of Diseases). It described the naked eye appearances in over 700 post-mortem examinations. The book by Wolff was *Theoria Generationis* (Theory of Generation). He supported epigenesis as against preformation in embryological development, and he set modern embryology on its way. Haemorrhage, the other major scourge of childbearing besides infection, was better understood because of the work of Edward Rigby (1747–1821) of Norwich. In 1775 he had published the *Essay on the Uterine Haemorrhage*. It made very little impact at the time but it was he who differentiated bleeding from the placental site in the lower part of the uterus (now placenta praevia) from that in the upper part. He wrote,

> 'There is no particular part of the Uterus, to which Nature seems constantly and uniformly to fix the Placenta. It is nevertheless, for the most part, so situated, that if the woman be healthy, and no accident befall her, it does not separate till the full term of pregnancy, nor then before the entire expulsion of the child, after which it becomes disengaged from the Uterus, and is thrown off, making room for its entire contraction, which shutting up the mouths of the vessels, effectually prevents any considerable loss of blood; for which purpose, it is plain it must be fixed to some part of the womb which does not dilate during labour, namely to the fundus or the sides of it. In this case, then, when a flooding comes on before the delivery of the child, it is obvious that the separation of the Placenta must be owing to some accidental circumstance ...'

Later he says,

> 'But from the uncertainty, with which ... Nature fixes the Placenta to the Uterus, it may happen to be so situated, that when the full term of pregnancy is arrived, and labour begins, a flooding necessarily accompanies it, and without the intervention of any of the above accidental circumstances; that is when it is fixed to the part of the womb which always dilates as labour advances ... That floodings, which arise from these two different causes, which I will distinguish by the names of accidental and unavoidable ... Of these two kinds of floodings, only one of them, namely, that which is produced by an accidental separation of the Placenta can be relieved by the use of these palliatives; and that the other, in which the Placenta is fixed to the Os Uteri, and the flooding is therefore unavoidable, cannot possibly be suppressed by any other method whatever, than the timely removal of the contents of the womb.'

The terms of 'accidental' and 'unavoidable' antepartum haemorrhage were in use for at least 150 years, being replaced by 'abruptio placentae' and 'placenta praevia' only in the second half of the 20th century. It is surprising that Rigby did not note that accidental haemorrhage is accompanied by pain, whereas unavoidable haemorrhage is not. But his general observations are correct, though the causes of accidental haemorrhage which he adduced, such as blows to the abdomen and so on, are not. It is interesting to note that he knew that the contractions of the upper uterus closed off the mouths of blood vessels and that emptying the uterus was the only way to stop bleeding.

The other major catastrophe – the fits of eclampsia – showed no signs of yielding to the understanding of the 18th century doctors or midwives. The treatment was still by bleeding and purging. It is possible that these might have had some effect on the reduction of cerebral oedema, but that pathology was not understood. It was simply that bleeding and purging were virtually routine for every variety of problem.

In about 1790 the birth rate in London surpassed that of the death rate. The population of England and Wales was then around eight million. The rise caused some anxiety and was expressed in 1798 by Thomas Malthus in his famous *Essay on the Principle of*

Population in which he enunciated the idea that rising populations would outgrow their food supplies. Another landmark for women in 1798 was Mary Wollstonecraft's *The Vindication of the Rights of Women.*

The Industrial Revolution is dated from about 1760. It caused an influx of people from the country to the towns where there were manufacturing industries. Women and children were used as sweated labour in the factories and coal mines. They were herded together in hovels in unhygienic conditions where infections were all too easily passed from one person to another. A result of poverty was malnutrition, causing short stature and small pelves. Women were ground down with work and childbearing. The prosperity of Britain and its increased population, on which so much depended for manual labour, was almost literally built on their tired aching backs.

CHAPTER NINE

Progress in the Nineteenth Century

With hindsight the essential problems of midwifery which had to be solved were those of:

1. Labour and the passage of the fetus through the birth canal.
2. Haemorrhage before and after birth.
3. Puerperal fever.
4. Convulsions, i.e. eclampsia.
5. Pain in labour and during operations.
6. Pregnancy and antenatal care.
7. The organization of the midwifery services.
8. Education and training of professionals.
9. The care of the baby.

It is probable that few people, if any, at the start of the 19th century saw the problems in the ways we do now. Each problem can only be solved when there is the understanding and the technology to deal with it. Until that time comes, the problems appear temporarily insuperable and it is only possible to get on and deal with what one can with the means available. So the emphases of the 19th century shifted from time to time. Progress in one area was accompanied by stagnation in others. Sometimes progress was on several fronts at once.

It is not surprising that for earlier midwives and doctors labour stood out as the most dramatic part of the whole reproductive process. It demanded attention in a way that the apparently quieter time of pregnancy did not. Moreover delivery could be seen to be a basically mechanical proceeding about which something could be done by the forceps or by internal version or at worst a destructive operation on the fetus. A further reason for concentration on delivery was that it was all too often a time of death for the mother and baby.

The mechanism of labour had been described during the 18th century by Ould and Smellie and by Solarés de Renhac (1737–1772) of Montpellier and Matthias Saxtorph (1740–1800) of Copenhagen. Midwifery had by then become of major interest to most of the western world. The rotations of the head and shoulders as they descended through the pelvis were well-known. There was knowledge of how to deal with various malpresentations, positions and lies, mainly by forceps and internal version in difficult labours.

Abdominal palpation had come to be used as an additional diagnostic aid to vaginal examination. This led to some definition of lie, presentation and position even before labour began. Vaginal examination was not needed to decide if the head or the breech presented. Moreover the fetal back could be felt and this gave an indication of the position of the occiput, with which it is in line. The position of the head in relation to the bony pelvis could therefore be known, i.e. occipito-anterior and occipito-posterior positions.

The diameters of the brim, cavity and outlet of the pelvis had been established. In general at the brim they were taken to be 4¼" antero-posteriorly, 4¾" diagonally and 5¼" transversely. For the cavity the average was 4¾" all round, while the outlet diameters were the reverse of those at the brim. These were thought to determine the mechanism of labour and the role of the soft parts of the pelvic floor musculature were at first ignored. Of course it was known that these average diameters could vary greatly and when they were small there was a contracted pelvis which might make delivery very difficult if not impossible.

However, Franz Karl Nägele (1777–1851) of Heidelberg in his *Mechanismus der Geburt* (Mechanism of Birth) of 1822 had described asynclitism which might overcome contraction at the brim naturally. He realized that the sacral promontory was at a higher level of the brim than the symphysis pubis. This meant that, when the head was transverse, one parietal eminence could slip past the promontory before the other one had negotiated its way past the pubis. In other words one eminence slipped into the cavity of the pelvis first and this made room for the other one to get in too by the head bending laterally. Since rickets often causes contraction of the brim, but often no other parts of the pelvis, this observation was very significant.

Arising from his interest in pelvic anatomy he described a rare anomaly in which one ala of the sacrum fails to develop, thus causing distortion and asymmetry of the pelvis and inability of the head to engage in the brim. Also in Germany F. Robert described, in 1842, an even rarer anomaly where both alae of the sacrum fail to develop. Because of the obvious importance of the size of the various parts of the pelvis attempts were made to measure it in life. Clinically this is very difficult. On vaginal examination some idea of general size can be obtained, but there can be no direct measurement of diameters, except at the outlet where bony points can be palpated. But the diameters that most, at that time, wanted to know were those of the brim. Some went so far as to put the whole hand in the vagina to try to measure it. The nearest to a direct measurement was to use the fingers to estimate the distance from the sacral promontory to the underside of the symphysis pubis – the so-called diagonal conjugate. An arbitrary three-quarters of an inch was deducted from this in the hope that this would be some more or less accurate measure of the antero-posterior diameter of the brim. But it was then the best available.

Jean Louis Baudelocque (1746–1810) of Paris, in 1789, had tried to overcome the problem of knowing the internal pelvic diameters by measuring between certain external bony points on the pelvis. He devised a caliper, called a pelvimeter, to make the measurements. The most important one, he thought, was that between the spine of the fifth lumbar vertebra and the top of the symphysis pubis. It became known as the external conjugate or Baudelocque's diameter. There were also measurements made between the anterior superior iliac spines, the great trochanters of the femur, the posterior superior iliac spines, and the iliac crests. Attempts were then made to relate all these to the internal measurements. They were in vogue for over a hundred years, but unfortunately they are quite useless. By 1851 Gustav Adolph Michaelis (1798–1848) of Kiel said so very firmly in his *Das Enge Becken* (The Female Pelvis). He analysed results in 72 cases and stated that, 'No importance must be attached to the distance between the crests of the ilium, and less still to that between the superior anterior spines.' He dismissed the other measurements too, but few seem to have taken his criticisms to heart despite their undoubted truth.

Michaelis discussed the causes of contracted pelvis and grouped them under the headings of rickets, heredity and length of legs. But he was patently honest in saying that, 'in the majority of nonrachitic pelvic cases, my enquiries yielded, on the whole, mostly negative results.' He described the rhomboid which bears his name. This is the area bounded by the spine of the fifth lumbar vertebra, the dimples over the two posterior superior iliac spines and the tip of the sacrum. If distorted it may show the absence of one or both sacral alae, or spondylolisthesis in which the body of the fifth lumbar vertebra slips forwards on the body of the first sacral vertebra.

Further investigation of the pelvis was by Carl Gustav Carus (1789–1869) of Dresden in 1820. He described the curve of the birth canal, now named after him. In mathematical terms he showed that the posterior wall of the birth canal is about 9" long and the front wall about 1¼" long. The canal is a cylinder which describes a forward bend. This was, of course, known to several earlier clinicians whenever they used the forceps but Carus delineated it more accurately than previously.

Many attempts were made to use these various understandings of the pelvis in forceps deliveries. The intention was always to mimic the natural processes as far as possible. There was comparatively little difficulty when the head was low in the pelvis. This problem had been virtually solved by Smellie and others like him. But when the head was high above the brim of the pelvis and would not engage, there were very great difficulties. First the cervix might not be fully dilated, and secondly inserting the blades of the forceps right up into the uterus is fraught with the danger of rupturing the uterus and maybe inability to grasp the fetal head safely. Nevertheless many obstetricians often made the attempt at 'high forceps'. This was because they could not with safety escape this dilemma by caesarean section. Their only alternative was perforation of the skull, evacuating the brain and pulling on the remains of the head with whatever tools they could devise. These developed into the cranioclast and cephalotribe which broke up the skull and then pulled on it. A cranioclast for breaking up the base of the skull was invented by James Young Simpson. He also produced a variety of forceps which became almost universally used.

To deal with the high head the operation of *accouchement forcée* was devised. There had to be manual dilatation of the cervix followed by application of the forceps to the head so that the baby could be forcibly pulled through the brim and down the pelvis to the exterior. But because of the lower forward curve of Carus it was difficult to pull the head in the right direction through the brim. It was in an attempt to deal with this problem that axis traction was devised.

Étienne Stéphane Tarnier (1828–1897) of Paris in 1877 designed traction rods which could be attached to ordinary curved forceps so that pull on the high head could be made to draw it accurately at right angles through the pelvic brim. W.C. Neville of Dublin in 1886 and Milne Murray of Edinburgh in 1891 produced similar devices for the same purpose. They were all intended to solve a problem of the times. Now delivery of the high head by forceps is no longer thought to be sufficiently safe for either mother or baby and it has therefore been abandoned, together with the devices.

The problem of the undilated cervix was addressed by Alfred Dührssen (1862–1933) of Berlin. In 1890 he advocated incising the cervix at 10, 2 and 6 o'clock when it would not dilate. In these positions it was unlikely to tear laterally at 3 and 9 o'clock into the broad ligament. Of course such incisions allowed for the application of forceps to the head. In fact using these incisions and delivering the baby by forceps came to be known as vaginal caesarean section. Unfortunately the incisions often did extend further than intended and there was often severe soft tissue damage as well. Yet such was the fear of caesarean section that this form of *accouchement forcée* was for a time acceptable.

The anxiety about disproportion and obstructed labour was so great that attempts were sometimes made to induce the onset of labour early to avoid having too large a baby. Thomas Denman of the Middlesex Hospital had advocated this in 1785, and later the same had been urged by Samuel Merriman (1771–1852) also of London in 1824. The operation, manually dilating the cervix and rupturing the membranes, was never widely adopted outside England. It often fails to achieve its purpose and is a potent way of introducing infection into the genital tract, though that was not understood until much later.

Other methods of induction included the insertion of stiff bougies through the cervix (Krause, 1853), not rupturing the membranes but stretching the lower uterine segment. Others inserted rubber bags though the cervix filling them with water by a tube running up to them. These were then pulled on in an effort to force the cervix open and start labour. The classic bag was that of Champetier de Ribes (1848–1935) described in 1888. They rarely worked and often burst.

The object of induction is to get the uterus to contract, and start labour. Ergot had been known for some time to do that. The credit for its therapeutic use goes to John Stearns (1770–1848) of New York. He wrote to a colleague about it in 1807 saying he had used the *pulvis parturiens* (parturient powder) for many years, especially because 'it expedites lingering parturition'. In 1822 Stearns wrote *Observations on Secale Cornutum*, or *Ergot, with directions for its use in Parturition*. He had collected the black grains of fungus (*Claviceps purpurea*) from infected rye grains and boiled half a drachm of this powder in half a pint of water 'and give one-third every twenty minutes until pains commence'. He also used a similar dose when labour was protracted; in inevitable abortion; when the placenta was retained after the birth of a baby; for haemorrhage after birth; for the prevention of haemorrhage by giving it just before the birth of a baby. In many ways this was all admirable advice, though giving ergot in the first stage of labour if there should be obstruction may cause rupture of the uterus.

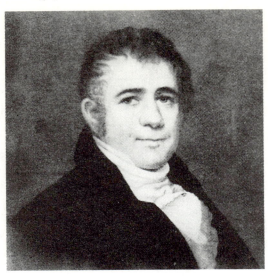

Fig. 9.1: Portrait of John Stearns

The problem with the use of liquid extract of ergot is that it contains very variable amounts of the active ingredients. Its action was therefore always uncertain. Moreover given by mouth it takes a long time for the effect to occur. Nevertheless this pioneer work showed that uterine contractions could be influenced pharmacologically, and later ecbolics, as they came to be called, have become a major part of the midwifery armamentarium. Samuel Merriman of London, in 1824, also wrote about ergot in his Synopsis of Difficult Labour, and so did J.H. Davis in his *Illustrations of Difficult Parturition*. The relative community of obstetric thought throughout the western world is once again demonstrated by these publications at roughly the same time.

Uterine contractions

There had come some appreciation of uterine contractions, especially in labour. But a fuller understanding of them came from Braxton Hicks (1823–1897) of Guy's Hospital in London. In 1872 he wrote *On the Contractions of the Uterus throughout Pregnancy*. He knew that contractions could be felt through the abdominal wall.

> 'The constancy with which these contractions of the uterus have always occurred to me leaves no doubt on my mind but that it is a natural condition of pregnancy irrespective of external irritation.'

It was a valuable independent sign of pregnancy.

> 'For the last six years and upwards I have made use of the intermittent action of the uterus as the principal symptom upon which I have depended in the diagnosis of pregnancy.'

The distinction between subjective symptoms and objective signs had not then been made. He went further. He knew that the contractions were not normally felt by the woman.

> 'Again, when the uterus has been excited by any cause, and these contractions are more than usually powerful, the woman is conscious of their presence, and by watching these we shall convince ourselves that the contractions, which were before unnoticed by her, are really the same as the so-called "pains" of premature expulsion of the foetus and also of true labour.'

> 'We need not, with the cognizance of this intermittent action, any longer wonder how it is that suddenly a new function is given to the uterus at the end of the ninth month; it is already in active exercise, not perceptible to the pregnant woman, though it is to the examining hand.'

This is magnificent clinical observation and deduction. The uterine muscle is active throughout reproductive life. And he made the crucial distinction between contractions and 'pains'. 'Pains' have remained a synonym for contractions for far too long. Contractions and the pain caused by them in labour require separate understanding for proper clinical management in the care of the patient.

Hicks realized that contractions were the cause of 'after-pains', the contractions sometimes felt in the puerperium, especially when a woman is breastfeeding. He observed too that contractions continued in pregnancy even when the baby was dead, and even when there was no baby as in hydatidiform mole.

Hicks guessed that the contractions aided the flow of blood through the placenta. Naturally he thought that they pumped the blood onwards, though later work shows that that is not true. Other mechanisms are at work.

More understanding of uterine muscle function came from Ludwig Bandl (1842–1892) latterly of Prague. He observed that when the uterus ruptured in obstructed labour the tear occurred in the lower part in what he called 'the thinned out cervix'. He was drawing attention to the fact that in labour there is a contracting upper part and a dilating more passive lower part. He described the ring of muscle which delineates the upper segment from the lower one when labour is obstructed. It is known as Bandl's ring or the retraction ring. It is recognizable clinically on inspection of the abdomen for the outline of the bladder can be seen. Its upper part is attached to the uterus at the point of union of the upper and lower segments. As the lower segment is stretched upwards it carries the bladder with it.

Operations for difficult labour

Forceps and internal version were the commonest operations used to cope with the problems of labour. *Accouchement forcée* and Dührssen's incisions have been noted. But among the commonest of the difficulties are malpositions and malpresentations. The malpositions are those of occipito-posterior and occipito-transverse where there is a failure of the occiput to rotate to come under the symphysis pubis. The ideal method of management in such cases is to rotate the head within the pelvis so that the occiput is brought to the front. It is easier said than done. Sometimes it can be achieved with the hand, though because of restrictions of space only the fingers and part of the palm can be used and not the thumb. Getting purchase on the head is the problem, for it is slippery and wet. The groove behind an ear may be of some help. Pulling on a shoulder by a hand on the abdomen may assist in rotating the body.

Despite the best efforts these attempts may fail. If the occiput is posterior it may be best simply to try to drag the baby out with the forceps as it lies. This may cause damage to both mother and baby. With the occipito-transverse this will not do. Forceps can be applied to the head, as older obstetricians often did, but this compresses the head because one blade is over the occiput and the other over the face, the worst possible application. In these circumstances it may be best to place the forceps blades correctly on the head with the blades over the ears, taking no notice for the time being that this is not a good application in conformity with the pelvis. It was, however, not a bad application when the straight-bladed forceps of Smellie were used, rather than those with a pelvic curve. With forceps applied correctly to the head it is of course possible to twist the forceps handles so that the occiput comes anterior. However, if that is done directly the forceps with a pelvic curve describe a wide arc inside the soft tissues of the cervix, vagina and musculature and are apt to lacerate them severely. To diminish this arc Friedrich Wilhelm Scanzoni (1821–1891) of Würzberg, near Frankfurt, devised his manoeuvre, in 1851, in which the handles outside the pelvis are swung in a wide arc centred in imagination on the tips of the blades of the forceps. Theoretically this causes minimal movement of the blades within the pelvis. No doubt this was true in the hands of the originator, but in others, less skilful, it was still damaging. With brow and face presentations, again manual manipulations were used in attempts to flex the head, or in the case of the face to rotate the chin to the front to allow delivery face to pubis. Forceps too might be used to draw the baby out.

When all else failed the only recourse was to perforate the skull, evacuate its contents to diminish its size and then pull out the head with a variety of instruments. Big shoulder diameters could be reduced by cleidotomy in which the clavicles were cut through with scissors.

Breech presentations were relatively easy to handle as they had been since Smellie's time and earlier. Groin traction, bringing down legs and arms and the application of forceps to the after-coming head were all within normal professional competence. Transverse lie in early labour was correctable by internal version. A variant on this was introduced by Braxton Hicks, who, in the 1860s, introduced *bipolar version*. This was possible when the cervix was only about 2–3 cms dilated. Two fingers were inserted through the cervix to push up the presenting part, then using abdominal manipulations the baby was turned until the fingers could catch hold of a foot and pull it down through the cervix. Then labour was allowed to proceed until full dilatation of the cervix when breech extraction could be performed.

Among the advantages claimed by Hicks for bipolar version was that it avoided the necessity for,

'The removal of the coat and the baring of the arm of the operator; and as a minor consideration the fatigue and pain endured by the operator while the hand is in the uterus.'

This gives a nice insight into the ways in which labour was conducted then.

For the neglected transverse lie, often with an arm delivered, the only recourse was decapitation. This was effected by scissors until Leonardo Gigli (1863–1908) of Florence produced his flexible wire saw in 1898. This could be passed round the neck which was then sawn through with comparative ease. The body could then be delivered by traction on the arm. The head came down afterwards as the uterus contracted and it could be pulled out either with forceps or some form of instrument attached to it.

Caesarean section

This operation was increasingly used later in the 19th century, mainly because of the advent of anaesthesia, which made it considerably less barbarous than it was previously. Yet it was still fraught with great danger of shock, haemorrhage and infection, any one of which could kill the patient. So it was used with great caution and circumspection.

Although drastic, a great step forward in prevention of fatal consequences was made by Edoardo Porro (1842–1902) of Pavia in Italy in a paper of 1876. In one of his cases he was unable to stem the bleeding from the incision in the uterus, so he performed subtotal hysterectomy and pulled the upper part of the amputated cervix, sutured and ligatured, into the lower part of the abdominal wound. This meant that the remains of the genital tract were isolated from the peritoneal cavity so that any infection of the cervical stump was on the surface and more easily dealt with. His patient recovered despite infection of the stump and urinary infection. The operation was performed under chloroform anaesthesia. In fact a similar operation had been carried out earlier by Horatio Robinson Storer of Boston, USA for a fibroid complicating pregnancy. Unfortunately his patient died on the third post-operative day. In the early 19th century the mortality of the operation was about 75 per cent. This new operation lowered that to about 50 per cent. By the end of the century the mortality had fallen to about ten per cent provided that section was done early in labour and before any other manipulations had been carried out.

Samuel Merriman in 1838 recorded only 13 survivals after 32 sections done in Great Britain. Collected cases from both Great Britain and the United States, from 1737–1858 showed maternal recovery in 23 cases out of 57 operations, 29 per cent. That is remarkable enough because it gives a recovery rate of almost 1 in 3, which modern professionals would scarcely have expected. Of course the Porro operation meant permanent sterility thereafter. He recognized a moral problem in this and consulted the bishop of Pavia who ruled that the operation was justified to save the life of the mother despite its resulting sterility. Another suggestion to make caesarean section safer was made by Philip Syng Physick (1768–1835) of Philadelphia in 1824. It was to approach the uterus without incising the peritoneum, i.e. an extra-peritoneal operation. It was technically difficult, especially in pre-anaesthetic days and was rarely done, despite the concept being an advanced one.

Delivery of the placenta

The third stage of labour tended to be conducted on the lines suggested by John Harvie, waiting for the abdominal signs of separation of the placenta, then using the contracted uterus as a sort of plunger to push the afterbirth out of the genital tract. Of course there were still those who used cord traction or proceeded immediately to manual removal. In an effort not to do this a method was devised by Carl Siegmund Credé (1819-1892) of Berlin in 1854. When the uterus did not separate the placenta from its walls, Credé gathered up the body of the uterus in both hands through the abdominal wall and then squeezed it hard to force the placenta out of the cavity. It perhaps had the merit of not invading the cavity with the hand, but it could still be very shocking and a cause of collapse of the patient.

Liquid extract of ergot came widely into use for trying to control the time of delivery of the placenta and prevent post-partum haemorrhage. It was variable in its efficacy for reasons mentioned previously.

Princess Charlotte and the management of labour

A case of British ultra-conservatism in the management of labour is shown by the tragic case of Princess Charlotte. She was the daughter of the Prince of Wales. He became regent when his father, George III, became incompetent through mental illness. He was later crowned as George IV. The Princess went into labour on 3rd November 1817 at the age of 21. Pregnancy had lasted 42 weeks. Her labour lasted two days and two nights. On 5th November she delivered a stillborn son weighing 9lb. This was followed by manual removal of placenta and there was an hour-glass constriction in the uterus which was confirmed at post-mortem. Five hours after the birth she became restless and died, possibly due to haemorrhage, shock or amniotic fluid embolus. She seems not to have lost much blood, but she did have breathlessness and pain in the chest. She had been attended by Sir Richard Croft, a physician-obstetrician. Although he knew the baby was big, at one time thinking there might be twins, he was reluctant to call in Dr Sims, who would have been able to apply the forceps. He was kept in an ante-room so that his presence should not distress the Princess. In a letter after the event Sims regretted that he had not been called upon by Croft. There was no doubt that they acted in accord with what was deemed to be the best practice. They were not blamed for their conduct by any members of the royal family. It preyed on the mind of Croft however to such an extent that he shot himself some time later.

The tragedy partly arose because of divided responsibilities and the belief of a physician that he knew best and was in command, using his lesser brethren as ancillaries. It seems to have been prevalent custom at the time. The historical significance is that if the stillborn baby had lived he would have been King. As it was, the death paved the way for Victoria to be crowned Queen in 1837.

Diagnosis

Of great importance was the discovery of the fetal heart sounds. In 1819 the Frenchman, René Laënnec (1781–1826) had first begun to listen to the adult heart through a tube applied to the chest. His pupil Jean Alexandre Lejumeau, Vicomte de Kergaredec

(1787–1877) first heard the fetal heart sounds. He wrote in 1822 *Mémoire sur l'auscultation appliqué à l'étude de la grossesse* (Memoir on auscultation as applied to the study of pregnancy). It was a discovery of some serendipity since with his tubular stethoscope he was hoping to hear the movements of the fetus. In 1830 Evory Kennedy of Dublin had heard the funic souffle, which arises when the stethoscope presses lightly on the umbilical cord, compressing it against some part of the fetal body. The soft swishing sound is in time with that of the fetal heart. The uterine souffle in time with the maternal pulse is due to the pressure of the stethoscope over the uterine vessels. It was sometimes thought to show where the placenta was situated but that is not true.

In 1837, William Fetherston Montgomery (1797–1859) of Dublin described the tubercles on the areolae of the breasts, which have ever after borne his name. His findings were in his *An Exposition of the Signs and Symptoms of Pregnancy*. In that book he described the breast changes of pregnancy at great length. He knew that the tubercles did not always completely regress in the multiparous patient.

In 1839 H.F. Nägele of Heidelberg drew attention to the fact that the fetal heart was usually maximally heard over the back, and therefore this gave some knowledge of the position of the baby's head within the pelvis, the back being in line with the occiput.

Abdominal examination was beginning to be used more frequently, though somewhat sporadically and not as a routine. Braxton Hicks, in 1872, as outlined earlier, knew that uterine contractions were virtually diagnostic of pregnancy, and that they could be felt by an examining hand on the abdomen. The sign could only be observed from about sixteen weeks of pregnancy onwards, when part of the uterus can be felt above the symphysis pubis.

In 1890 Christian Gerhard Leopold (1846–1912), with M.E.C. Pantzer, described four manoeuvres of abdominal palpation, which are much like those used since. These authors amplified work on the subject by Carl Credé (1819–1892) and Adolph Pinard (1844–1934), the latter being the inventor of the well-known trumpet shaped fetal stethoscope. It is surprising now to realize how comparatively late in the development of midwifery abdominal palpation came to be used and accepted. James Read Chadwick (1844–1905) of Boston, USA described the colour of the vagina in pregnancy in 1877.

> 'The color begins as a pale violet in the early months, becomes more bluish as pregnancy advances, until it often assumes finally a dusky, almost black, tint; this last is familiar to every obstetrician.'

Then Alfred Hegar (1830–1914) of Freiberg in Germany described his sign for the diagnosis of early pregnancy. It was publicized in a paper of 1884, by Hegar's pupil, C. Reinl. It was called *A Positive Symptom for the Diagnosis of Pregnancy in the First Months*. Hegar himself wrote about his sign later in 1895. On vaginal examination he found the cervix to be soft, the upper part of the uterus globular and mobile, on a lower segment that was scarcely palpable. In favourable cases the diagnosis of pregnancy could be made at six or seven weeks.

Albuminuria

An event of subsequent great significance was the discovery in 1843, by John Charles Weaver Lever (1811–1858) of Guy's Hospital, that albumin was found in the urine of patients who had had convulsions (eclampsia) in pregnancy or the puerperium. The finding of albumin in the urine had been first described by Richard Bright (1789–1858) in kidney diseases which for long were named after him. He was a Guy's physician too. Lever did the tests because he thought that there were similarities between eclampsia and Bright's Disease. He thought therefore that eclampsia was a form of renal disease. Up to a point that is true but not exactly so. Extending his observations he found that albuminuria often occurred in those women who had premonitory symptoms of eclampsia, such as headaches, oedema, blurred vision and a sensation of flashing lights. Fits were liable to follow later. Despite this new knowledge there were still no efficacious forms of treatment.

All these findings began to suggest that there were important things to discover about pregnancy, which had previously been largely ignored. Pregnant women, up to then, were rarely examined physically. Their condition was deemed to be a natural one which could largely take care of itself, unless there was some catastrophe such as fits or bleeding. The upper classes were advised on diet which was usually bland and they were enjoined to rest. Poorer folk were not seen at all until they went into labour.

Expected date of delivery

This was well known to occur around ten lunar months or nine calendar months plus seven days from the first day of the last menstrual period. This was known as Nägele's Rule. Within limits it is fairly satisfactory. It puts the average length of pregnancy at about 280 days. But, of course, the true length of pregnancy is from the day of fertilization to the birth. It is now known that ovulation is usually about 14 days before the succeeding period. In a 28-day cycle that is of course also 14 days after the preceding period, but in a 35 day cycle ovulation is 21 days after the previous period begins. The day of ovulation is also about the time of fertilization and the fertilization to delivery interval is therefore about 266 days.

None of this was known in the 19th century, the time of ovulation often being thought to be just after the period or just before the next one. Naturally this led to some confusion. Yet the duration of pregnancy was of some importance, especially where matters of inheritance of wealth and title were concerned and where there might have been doubt about who was the father of a child.

In 1816 five obstetricians for the House of Lords decided that no pregnancy could last beyond 40 weeks. But later James Young Simpson averred that it could last longer and cited instances from his own practice where pregnancy had lasted between 319 and 365 days. This last may be excessive. Yet some women may have prolonged absence of periods before they become pregnant. They could therefore then have been deemed to have long gestations when, in fact, they had only had long periods of amenorrhoea, during only 266 days (or thereabouts) of which they had been pregnant. This possibility was not recognised until the 20th century.

Haemorrhages

These were known, as they still are as (a) antepartum, i.e. accidental and unavoidable, and (b) post-partum, after the delivery of the baby. Rigby in 1775 had correctly discerned the two varieties of antepartum haemorrhage, but there was only slow acceptance of his ideas, perhaps because there was relatively little that could be done about either of them, or maybe that they now seemed to be obvious.

For accidental haemorrhage and for unavoidable haemorrhage (placenta praevia) the vagina was often stuffed very tightly with cloth packings of many kinds. Binders were applied to the abdomen too. Liquid extract of ergot was given by mouth. There must have been only limited success with these methods. Possibly in unavoidable haemorrhage the pack would compress the placenta between it and the fetal head. In accidental haemorrhage, where the placenta is in the upper part of the uterus a pack was probably futile, except that it might cause uterine contractions so being a form of induction of labour.

For a long time it had been usual to treat both forms of antepartum haemorrhage by internal version and delivery. Delivery of both baby and placenta is, of course, the only certain way of stopping the bleeding as the uterus contracts down firmly on the blood vessels in the placental bed. In many cases of unavoidable haemorrhage, in order to be able to perform the operation the hand had to be thrust through the placenta, so the bleeding is increased.

Strangely, even such an eminent obstetrician as James Young Simpson thought that the bleeding came from the placenta itself, rather than from its bed and maternal blood vessels. Because of this he advocated, in accidental haemorrhage, that the placenta should be manually separated from the uterine wall. This shows that there was still great ignorance about the maternal and fetal circulations of the placenta.

Induction of labour by rupturing the membranes could, of course, have some success. In unavoidable haemorrhage the presenting part might then be pressed down on the placenta by the uterine contractions and so diminish bleeding. Induction was also probably valuable in accidental haemorrhage if the woman went into labour and delivered both baby and placenta fairly rapidly. Moreover it came to be realized that there were two forms of accidental haemorrhage, 'revealed' which was comparatively mild in its effects on the patient, and 'concealed', which was severe, causing much pain and shock.

Even better was the case where the breech presented. A leg could then be brought down, and when pulled on it would exert pressure through the baby's bottom pressing on the placental bed in unavoidable haemorrhage. This became known as 'plugging with the half breech'. It became the preferred method after Braxton Hicks had described 'bipolar version'. This was especially valuable since it could be performed, with two fingers rather than the whole hand, before full dilatation of the cervix. The alternative of internal version, which was frequently used, required forcible dilatation of the cervix in order to get the hand right inside the cavity of the uterus.

Towards the end of the century when anaesthesia was increasingly available it became possible to perform caesarean section. Lawson Tait (1845–1899) of Birmingham, England, is credited with the first such operation for placenta praevia, done in 1898. It was of course a Porro caesarean hysterectomy.

One can only imagine now how helpless everyone must have felt in the face of these severer antepartum haemorrhages. All the available remedies were fearful and frightful and of doubtful outcome. Even towards the end of the century the maternal mortality for placenta praevia was 30 per cent and the fetal mortality 60 per cent. These obviously included the milder cases, so in the more severe ones the mortality must have been dreadful. The same must have been true for accidental haemorrhage too. There were no means of resuscitation by blood transfusion. Even worse it was not uncommon to bleed the patient as a therapeutic measure. Often all forms of haemorrhage were thought to be due to plethora on the assumption that the organs were stuffed with blood, and that that was the cause of haemorrhage.

Post-partum haemorrhage

In perhaps about 90 per cent of labours there was comparatively little bleeding in the third stage of labour. The placenta separates from its bed almost as soon as the baby is delivered. It then drops into the lower segment of the uterus or the vagina from where it can easily be expelled by the manoeuvre of using the contracted uterus in the abdomen as a plunger, described by John Harvie. The empty uterus then contracts down and so controls the vessels of the placental bed.

However in about ten per cent of deliveries there may be severe bleeding either before or after delivery of the placenta. If before it may be that the haemorrhage is due to only partial separation of the placenta from the uterine wall. The vessels in its bed can then bleed freely because the uterus cannot contract properly to close them off. The treatment must obviously be manual removal of the placenta. The professionals of the 19th century undertook this with much less reluctance than later. For some of them it was virtually routine to perform the operation.

After delivery of the placenta many obstetricians attempted to pack the uterus and vagina with long lengths of linen bandages. It must have been extremely difficult before the coming of anaesthesia. Yet apart from the pressure exerted by the pack it might have induced firm contraction of the uterine musculature in some cases. Obviously liquid extract of ergot was given too to bring on contractions, but it was unreliable because the active ingredients were so variable in quantity in the solution, and because there was a delay of up to half an hour before any of them could reach the uterus, since the preparation had to be given by mouth.

There was no knowledge then of the bleeding disorders which can follow labour, and which can seem to be unstoppable without modern technology. And of course there was no blood transfusion.

Puerperal fever

The scene had been set for the understanding of the nature of puerperal fever by Charles White in 1773 and by Alexander Gordon in 1795. Gordon especially had come to know that something was carried from patient to patient by attendants at births. His evidence was conclusive but the midwifery establishment refused to accept it, and hounded him for his then unorthodox views. Both doctors were concerned with forms of disinfection, with personal cleanliness of midwives and doctors, with ventilation and isolation of patients. They were at a loss to understand just what it was that was being conveyed to patients but they were· groping for a method of prevention transmission of infection.

In Vienna, Ignaz Philipp Semmelweis (1818–1865) was appointed to the First Obstetric Clinic in 1844. He was ousted from this post and joined instead the department of pathology, under the direction of the renowned Carl Rokitansky (1804-1878). Semmelweis observed that the mortality from puerperal fever was very much greater in that part of the hospital where medical students attended the women in labour than in the part where women were attended by midwives. He noted that students attended post-mortem examinations, often on infected patients, whereas the midwives did not. The students would often proceed straight from the autopsy room to the labour wards, there to perform vaginal examinations with their bare hands. For teaching purposes each woman had to undergo several such examinations. The women of Vienna knew and feared all this and always did their utmost not to go into the student section. They left delivery to the very last moment so that they would be taken to the midwives' part of the hospital.

Semmelweis had a male friend who had died after cutting his finger when doing an autopsy. He saw that the illness preceding the death was very similar to that of the clinical course of puerperal fever.

Semmelweis made his observations during the years 1841–1846. The mortality from fever was often as high as 9.9 per cent. There must have been many more who later suffered from chronic pelvic sepsis. In 1847 he instituted a regime which he insisted that all students should follow. It consisted essentially of thorough scrubbing of the hands and then rinsing them with chloride of lime as a disinfectant. The results were almost miraculous. In 1846 the mortality was 11.8 per cent. In the two following years, just after the regime was introduced, it was 3.8 per cent and 1.27 per cent respectively. This last was even better than that of 1.33 per cent in the midwives' section. He wrote,

> 'Puerperal Fever is caused by conveyance to the pregnant woman of putrid particles derived from living organisms, through the agency of the examining fingers.'

This showed incredible insight, for the science of bacteriology had not yet begun.

His work convinced his own chiefs, including Rokitansky, and further afield great figures like Hegar and Michaelis. But others, among them Carl Braun the Professor of Obstetrics in Vienna, refused to accept it. They blamed the weather for the epidemics.

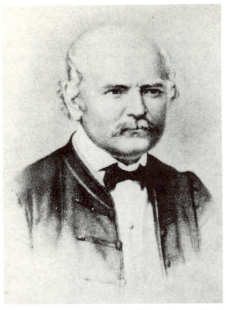

Fig. 9.2: Portrait of Ignaz Philipp Semmelweiss

Semmelweis then showed that this was not true by comparing meteorological records with those of the incidence of fever. They also said that those who suffered from the fever were 'the most loose and abandoned in the community'. They blamed wounded modesty since women were examined by male students. Could the women be both loose and modest? Another canard perpetrated by them was that the fever was conveyed by the sperm. Semmelweis pointed out that all pregnancies were started by sperm in whichever part of the hospital the women were delivered.

Not surprisingly Semmelweis left Vienna in high dudgeon because of the hostile reception of his ideas. In 1855 he was appointed Professor of Obstetrics in his native Budapest. Despite his aversion to writing, in 1861 he published his classic *Die Aetiologie, der Begriff und die Prophylaxis des Kindbettfiebers* (The Aetiology, Course and Prophylaxis of Childbed Fever). In the same year he published *Open Letters to Sundry Professors of Obstetrics* in which he roundly castigated his critics.

By 1863 he suffered from manic-depressive attacks, perhaps partly because of the adversities he had undergone. He had to be admitted to a mental hospital. He died there, 15 days after admission, of an infection contracted while he was operating on a gynaecological patient. He is one of the most tragic figures in the history of midwifery.

In America there was a happier tale to tell. Oliver Wendell Holmes (1809–1894) was Professor of Anatomy and Physiology at Harvard in Boston, Massachusetts from 1847 to 1882, and he became Dean of the Faculty. Before that he had practised in the city. He was also a towering literary figure, with obviously a superb command of English. His major work was *The Autocrat at the Breakfast Table*. He was a most considerable figure in his community, and carried much weight there.

In 1843 Holmes gave a lecture to the Boston Society for Medical Improvement. He had previously observed a colleague who had cut himself during the conduct of a post-mortem examination on a woman who had died of puerperal fever. The colleague died a week later. Before doing the autopsy several of his patients had contracted puerperal fever. The lecture was published in the *New England Quarterly Journal of Medicine* which was not widely read and it ceased publication after only one year. The essay was published again in 1855 when it was called *Puerperal Fever as a Private Pestilence*. We would probably interpret 'Private Pestilence' as being an epidemic occurring in a particular doctor's practice.

Holmes was trenchant.

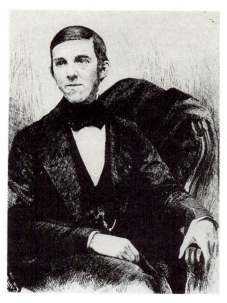

Fig. 9.3: Portrait of Oliver Wendell Holmes

'The practical point to be illustrated is the following: The disease known as puerperal fever is so far contagious as to be frequently carried from patient to patient by physicians and nurses.'

and,

'... that whenever and wherever they can be shown to carry disease and death instead of health and safety, the common instincts of humanity will silence every attempt to explain away their responsibility.'

Like Gordon he caused a furore among other doctors and midwives. He drew the conclusions that a physician should not take any active part in the conduct of an autopsy on a woman dying of puerperal fever; if he should do so he should thoroughly clean himself and his clothing; he should do the same if he attended a case of erysipelas. If a case of puerperal fever should occur in his practice he should not undertake further deliveries for some weeks, preferably a month. If the doctor should have three or more cases of the fever in his practice then that was *prima facie* evidence that he was a carrier of the disease. He said,

'... the time has come when the existence of a private pestilence in the sphere of a single physician should be looked upon, not as a misfortune, but a crime: and in the knowledge of such occurrence the duties of the practitioner to his profession should give way to his paramount obligations to society.'

There was much more in this vein.

A formidable opponent of these views was Charles D. Meigs (1792–1869), Professor of Obstetrics and Gynaecology at Jefferson College, Philadelphia, who was incensed by the thought that a gentleman's hands might not be clean. He drew attention to the fact that cases had even occurred in the practice of James Young Simpson in Edinburgh. Holmes delivered one of the most withering counterblasts in the history of obstetrics to this.

'I take no offence and attempt no retort. No man can quarrel with me over the counterpane that covers a mother with her newborn infant at her breast.'

and,

'Dr Simpson attended the dissection of two of Dr Sydney's cases and freely handled the dissected parts. His next four childbed patients were affected with puerperal fever and it was the first time he had seen it in his practice. As Dr Simpson is a gentleman [Dr Meigs as above], and as a gentleman's hands are clean [Dr Meigs as above], it follows that a gentleman with clean hands may carry the disease.'

Professor Meigs was still not convinced as he should have been.

Holmes seems not to have heard of White, Gordon or even his contemporary Semmelweis, though he does refer to one 'Senderein', which may be a misunderstanding of the name. It would appear that many were on the same track though making their discoveries independently.

Joseph Lister (1827–1912) graduated from London University in 1852. It was at University College Hospital that he witnessed the first operation under anaesthesia in England. The surgeon was Robert Liston who hailed from Edinburgh. There was then a strong Scottish influence in London. Lister was advised to further his education in Edinburgh under the tutelage of the famous James Syme, whose daughter he subsequently married. In 1860 he was elected Professor of Surgery in Glasgow.

Lister was disturbed to note that the mortality in his cases of amputation was 45 per cent, mainly due to sepsis. The discharge from such wounds was then known as 'laudable pus'. In 1865 the Professor of Chemistry in Glasgow drew Lister's attention to the work of Louis Pasteur (also a chemist) in France. He was the virtual founder of the science of bacteriology. Lister realized that septic wounds might be due to bacteria similar to those demonstrated by Pasteur.

Pasteur had shown that bacteria could be destroyed by heat but this was inapplicable in clinical practice. Lister therefore sought chemical antiseptics. He tried several but then lighted on carbolic acid or phenol. He used this for dressing compound fractures where the skin was broken. The results were virtually miraculous. He published a series of papers in the Lancet in 1867 and the principles of antisepsis were established. He extended the use of phenol in his famed 'carbolic spray', where phenol was vaporized in the operating theatres of the day.

In 1877 Lister moved to King's College Hospital in London. There was still then no great use of antiseptics in midwifery. A few, such as Lombe Atthill in Dublin insisted by 1875 that all students and midwives should scrub their hands with carbolic soap and then rinse them in carbolic acid before attending women in childbed. By 1881 Étienne Tarnier in Paris was using carbolic acid in midwifery.

It was through the General Lying-in Hospital, York Road, Lambeth, that Lister came to have a major impact on midwifery. It was only two or three miles away from King's College Hospital. The lay governors of the Lying-in Hospital recorded in 1878,

> 'The death rate during the year has been unfortunately very high, and as towards the end of the year [1877] it did not appear to decrease it was deemed advisable to close the hospital for a time and to thoroughly cleanse the House and let the repairs proceed.'

The deaths were mainly due to puerperal fever. The hospital remained closed for almost two years. From 1833 to 1860 the maternal mortality from the fever had been 30.8 per thousand. It fell to 17 per 1,000 between 1861 and 1877, but then rose to 53 per 1,000 just before the closure.

The treatment of these cases, by younger members of the staff, had been by putting the patients in ice baths and douching the interior of the uterus with various medicaments. This angered several of the older doctors and midwives and the quarrel caused much dissension and led finally to several of the staff resigning or being sacked.

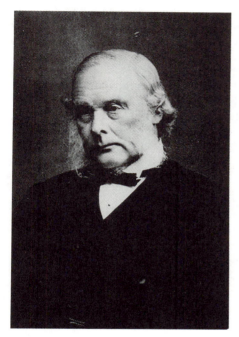

Fig. 9.4: Portrait of Lord Lister of antisepsis fame

Significantly, however, on 4th December 1878 the governors decided to appoint 'Joseph Lister Esq., FRS, to be Consulting Surgeon to this Hospital'. He obviously introduced antiseptic principles into midwifery. This was very important since the General Lying-in Hospital was one of the most important places for the training of midwives, and they travelled far and wide when they left, taking the Listerian antiseptic principles with them.

Just after the hospital re-opened in 1880 there were 230 in-patients, three of whom died but only one of puerperal sepsis. In 1881 there were 281 in-patients and 726 out-patients and there were no deaths. This was a fantastic turnaround. The governors recorded 'Antiseptic treatment has been adopted in all cases and the results have fully justified our expectations'. It is interesting to note too that by 1894 the staff were regularly measuring the temperatures of patients with thermometers. Prior to this estimates of fever were made on the appearance of the patient and feeling the warmth of the skin. The clinical thermometer had been brought into practice by Sir Clifford Allbutt of Leeds in 1867.

It is pleasing to note that Lister was made a baronet in 1883 and was raised to the peerage in 1897, the first medical man to be so honoured. In January of that year he accepted the invitation to become President of the General Lying-in Hospital, and he remained so until his death in 1912. He undoubtedly influenced midwifery practice very greatly through his direct association with the Hospital, and that is not sufficiently widely known.

It was not until 1884 that Lister acknowledged the work of Semmelweis, of whom he had heard only in that year. It is now surprising that so little was known of pioneer work going on in other centres. The key to all the previous attempts at understanding the nature of puerperal fever was, of course, bacteriology. The most important figure of the time was Louis Pasteur (1822–1895). In 1874 Lister had written to him to say how valuable his work had been in helping to introduce antisepsis. Pasteur was one of the greatest scientists of all time and his work ranged far and wide. But for the good of midwifery he and his pupils found bacteria in the blood and lochia of a woman who died of puerperal fever. At a meeting of the Academy of Medicine in Paris, Pasteur interrupted a lecture on puerperal fever, saying,

> 'None of these things cause the epidemic. It is the nursing and medical staff who carry the microbe from an infected woman to a healthy one'.

He drew a series of dots on the blackboard and said that this microbe *en chapelet de grains* was the cause. They were, of course, streptococci, the main infecting organism of puerperal fever then.

It had taken something over a hundred years, from Charles White's time, to get to this stage of the understanding of the nature of puerperal fever. It had been a scourge and pestilence of childbearing women since the dawn of time. For the first time at the end of the 19th century there came the possibility that its causes could be known and therefore that it could be prevented and at a later date cured.

Anaesthesia

Pain had always been thought to be an inevitable part of labour. 'In sorrow thou shalt bring forth' said the Bible, or in a later translation 'with pain will you give birth to children'. It was the curse of Eve. It was accepted in christian societies as God's will for nearly 2,000 years. No doubt many analgesics had been given to women, over the centuries, to relieve the pains of labour. Perhaps these included opium, mandrake, henbane, cannabis and alcohol. But almost nowhere in the older literature of midwifery is there reference to attempts to relieve pain in labour or during the terrifying ordeals of the operations of midwifery.

Several anaesthetics were known before the 19th century but had not been used as such, even in surgery. 'Sweet vitriol' was known in Spain in the 13th century. It was made by mixing oil of wine (alcohol) with spirits of vitriol (sulphuric acid). The result was crude ether.

In 1772 Joseph Priestley (1733–1804) discovered 'laughing gas' or nitrous oxide. It was used at house parties to bring on mild intoxication. In 1799 Humphry Davy (1778–1829), of miner's lamp fame, inhaled nitrous oxide and tried it out on several men, and emphasized its pleasurable qualities. In 1800 he wrote about it and said,

> 'As nitrous oxide in its extensive operation appears capable of destroying physical pain, it may probably be used with advantage during surgical operations in which no great effusion of blood takes place ...',

but this idea was not then followed up.

Michael Faraday (1791–1867), renowned for his work on electricity, about 1818 made a study of ether. He wrote,

'When the vapour of ether, mixed with common air, is inhaled it produces effects very similar to those occasioned by nitrous oxide. By the incautious breathing of ether vapour, a man was thrown into a lethargic condition, which, with a few interruptions, lasted for thirty hours'.

Again this was not followed up, and ether continued to be used for 'ether frolics' at social gatherings, for its mild intoxicating effects.

Chloroform was discovered in 1831 in several countries and its composition ($CHCl_3$) was known by 1835, but its anaesthetic properties were not investigated.

The first deliberate use of ether as an anaesthetic was probably by Crawford Williamson Long, of Jefferson, Georgia, USA, when he removed a cyst from the back of a colleague in 1842. He published nothing about it until much later.

In 1844 in Hartford, Connecticut, a medical student, Gardner Colton, gave stage shows of laughing gas in which he induced members of the audience to inhale nitrous oxide to experience its hilarious effects. One person stumbled against a settee and bruised himself severely, but made no complaint. Horace Wells, a dentist, witnessed this and realized the potential value of laughing gas in his practice. He invited young Colton to come to his surgery the next day, equipped to give gas for a tooth extraction. The patient was Wells himself. The tooth was pulled out and Wells felt no pain. He tested it out on several patients who also felt no pain. Excited by his successes Wells went to Boston, Mass. to tell his erstwhile partner, Thomas Green Morton. He knew John Collins Warren the famous surgeon of the Massachusetts General Hospital. He was persuaded to allow Wells to administer the gas during an operation. It was an ignominious failure in this case.

Morton, however, persisted, with the idea of the relief of pain and lighted on ether. With the aid of a chemist, Charles T. Jackson the ether was purified and used successfully. He returned to John Collins Warren and persuaded him once more, on 30th September 1846, to experiment, this time with ether. A vascular tumour of the jaw was excised and the patient felt no pain. Warren said, 'A new era has opened on the operating surgeon'. (It promised to be of value to patients too!)

There was some unseemly wrangling between Morton and Jackson about patenting ether, so that each might make money out of it, but fortunately this disreputable episode was soon over. Ether quickly became known and used in many parts of the world. On 21st November 1846 Oliver Wendell Holmes wrote to Morton and suggested that the state induced by ether should be called 'anaesthesia', signifying insensibility, and the adjective should be 'anaesthetic'. Those terms have been used ever since.

A witness of this first operation by Warren was Jacob Bigelow, Professor of Surgery at Harvard. On 28th November 1846 he wrote to a friend, Dr James Boott, of Gower Street in London. He was a native of Boston. Bigelow said,

'I send you an account of a new anodyne process lately introduced here, which promises to be one of the important discoveries of the present age. It has rendered many patients insensible to pain during surgical operations, and other causes of suffering.'

Boott used ether very quickly on a patient with toothache. He told Robert Liston, surgeon of University College Hospital, about this new discovery. Liston hurried round to Peter Squire, a chemist in Oxford Street, to have him make ether. The chemist tried it out on his nephew. On 21st December the Squires gave ether to a man about to have an amputation done by Liston. He felt nothing and fell back in a faint after the operation when he found it had been completed.

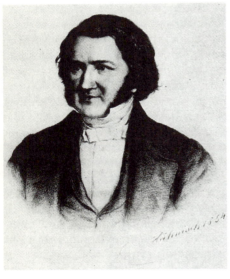

Fig. 9.5: Portrait of James Young Simpson of Edinburgh

James Young Simpson (1811–1870), who had been appointed to the Chair of Midwifery in Edinburgh in 1840, was on a Christmas holiday in London in 1846, with his friend Robert Liston from whom he learned about ether. By November 1847 Simpson had been using ether in midwifery for about ten months, so he had wasted no time putting what he had learned into practice. About the same time Dr Walter Channing, Professor of Obstetrics at Harvard, had been using it. He was probably the first to do so in midwifery since he was on the spot in Boston, Massachusetts, where ether was first used. Of course administration was by the old 'rag and bottle' method in which the ether was dripped from a bottle on to a cloth over the patient's mouth and nose. It came to be known later as 'open ether'.

Simpson was a man of insatiable energy, experimenting, thinking and writing on a variety of subjects, not always medical, or obstetric and gynaecological. He was not fully content with ether. It had an unpleasant clinging smell; it made many patients sick; it irritated the eyes and it had a tendency to catch fire. It has to be remembered that most deliveries were conducted in private homes with open fires in the bedrooms, as well as candles or paraffin lamps for lighting, and later coal gas. He thought there must be more suitable substances which could be used as anaesthetics. He tried out many chemicals on himself and his friends and assistants, often after dinner at his home at 52, Queen Street. This, of course, was potentially very dangerous. On at least two occasions Mrs Simpson found her husband unconscious on the floor of the basement of his home where he often worked on sniffing a variety of substances to discover anaesthetic effects.

The lucky break came when David Waldie, a chemist working in Liverpool, but an old friend of Simpson's, visited him. Waldie suggested that chloroform might be tried.

Simpson had some made by Duncan and Flockhart, the chemists of Edinburgh. He did not think it looked promising so laid it aside. But Matthews Duncan, a friend and colleague had tried it out in the laboratory of Dr Gregory in the University. He told Simpson about it.

On 4th November 1847 Simpson with Duncan and other friends were at the table after dinner and started their sniffings. Then Simpson remembered his bottle of chloroform, which he retrieved from under a pile of waste paper. The doctors put the chloroform in tumblers and began to sniff. A record of the time says,

> 'Immediately an unwonted hilarity seized the party; they became bright eyed, very happy, and very loquacious, expatiating on the delicious aroma of the new fluid.'

Conversation flowed freely and the ladies were delighted by it, but then proceedings were rudely interrupted as each of the three doctors crashed to the floor. When they recovered they and the ladies continued to sniff the chloroform until it was all gone. It was in this improbable way, on a cold November night, that one of the great revolutions in midwifery practice came about. Pain could be banished from the worst experiences of childbirth and the necessary operations consequent upon it. It is not surprising that euphoria prevailed, though time had to pass before the drawbacks of chloroform came to be known, and better methods of anaesthesia could be devised.

There were many people who objected to the relief of pain in labour, especially clergymen. Doctors said chloroform would increase the number of deaths. Statistics gathered by Simpson showed that this was not true. The clerics quoted Genesis over and over again, reminding of the curse of Eve, that there ought to be pain in labour. Simpson was equal to this. He pointed out that God had put Adam to sleep to remove a rib out of which Eve was fashioned. God was the first anaesthetist! He pointed out that there were many instances of interference with the natural order as in clothing, transport and much else of civilized living.

The criticisms of the use of chloroform to relieve the pains of labour were largely silenced when Queen Victoria accepted its use for that purpose on 7th April 1853 at the birth of Prince Leopold. It was administered by Dr John Snow (1815–1858). She had the anaesthetic again in 1857 at the birth of Princess Beatrice. For many years afterwards this was known as administering chloroform *à la reine*. The Queen was head of the Church of England and a devout christian, carrying immense moral authority. Chloroform came to be used around the world in midwifery and surgery. All became convinced of its undoubted value.

Simpson was a great figure in midwifery and the wider world of his time. He improved the obstetric forceps. He invented a suction tractor which might be used to apply to the fetal scalp in order to draw the head out of the pelvis. It was not a success but it foreshadowed another more effective instrument of the 20th century. At first he rejected the work of Semmelweis on puerperal fever, but later embraced it. He was erroneous in manually separating the placenta from the uterine wall in cases of accidental haemorrhage in the belief that the bleeding came from the placenta itself. But his more positive contributions were massive and lasting.

In 1866 he was made a baronet. He was a moving spirit in setting up the General Medical Council for Registration and Education, to control the training and education of doctors in the United Kingdom. At his funeral on 13th May 1870 crowds lined the streets of Edinburgh and brought the city to a virtual standstill, such being the popular esteem in which he was held. He was known to be a man who had helped to banish much of the intolerable anguish and pain of childbirth and surgery. Through his work he was a major benefactor of all mankind.

A slighter advance on the administration of chloroform was made by Ferdinand E. Junker who invented a special inhaler in 1867. Air was blown by a hand bulb through the liquid which was vaporized and carried through a tube to a metal mask, with lint stretched over it. The mask was deliberately ill-fitting to the nose and mouth so that excess of the anaesthetic could not build up. It remained in use until the middle of the 20th century.

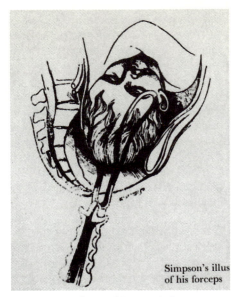

Simpson's illus of his forceps

Fig. 9.6: Use of Simpson's forceps

Some scientific advances

In 1824 two Frenchmen, Jean Louis Prévost (1790–1850) and Jean Baptiste André Dumas (1800–1884) had shown that fertilization in the frog was due to the entry of a spermatozoon into the egg. In 1827 Ernst von Baer (1792–1876) of Germany first saw a mammalian ovum, that of a bitch. He made extensive studies of embryology and established that the embryo developed from the three primary germ layers of ectoderm, mesoderm and endoderm. This finally destroyed preformationism in favour of epigenesis. Johannes Müller (1801–1858) of Germany in 1830 described the embryological development of the uterus from the Müllerian ducts, and clearly depicted the mesonephric remnants in the broad ligaments.

From 1841 to 1854 Robert Lee (1793–1877) of St George's Hospital, London, investigated the anatomy of the sympathetic nerve supply of the uterus, and lectured upon it in 1841. This was followed up, 25 years later, with further investigation by Ferdinand Frankenhäuser (1832–1894), Professor at Zürich. The exact role of these nerves is still something of a mystery. Theodor Langhans (1839–1915) of Germany in 1877 defined the cell layer of the placenta, ever since named after him.

The rise of bacteriology had much later significance for midwifery, and indeed of all medicine. Little could be done about the treatment and cure of many infections, but the scene was being set for that to be done. The organism of gonorrhoea was described in 1879. That of tuberculosis in 1882. In fact 21 new pathogenic bacteria were characterised between 1879 and 1900. The common infecting organism of the urinary tract, *Escherischia Coli* was discovered in 1885, when it was called *Bacterium coli commune* because it was often found in the colon.

Attempts at treatment of infections was by making vaccines. These are attenuated organisms which when administered may excite immune responses which can protect the patient. Such vaccination was used by Edward Jenner (1749–1823) against smallpox in 1798. Louis Pasteur vaccinated a boy against rabies in 1885, and the experiment was successful. Emil von Behring (1854–1917) in 1891 prepared an antitoxin against diphtheria which protected against the disease.

Scientific thought, especially of biology, was revolutionized in the second half of the 19th century by the publication of Charles Darwin's (1809–1882) *On The Origin of the Species by means of Natural Selection* published in 1859. From this point onwards the way of looking at all living phenomena changed, almost beyond recognition, from what had been thought before. The change did not, of course, come about abruptly but it has gradually come to dominate all biological science, including that of medicine.

Education and training

Through many centuries there had been sporadic attempts to educate and train doctors and midwives. There had been the famous School of Salerno in the 13th century. William Smellie and John Leake in London had schools of midwifery expressly for the education and training of both midwives and doctors in the 18th century. The courses comprised a series of lectures with practical work in delivery. At the end of the course a certificate was granted to show some sort of qualification. Rather isolated from one another, there were similar schools in Edinburgh, Paris, Dublin and Philadelphia and elsewhere.

The various schools constructed their own curricula. There was no overall consensus on what should be taught and for how long, and by whom. The value of the certification must have been very variable. There had, of course, been some indifferent control of the quality of the practice of physicians, surgeons and apothecaries. The Royal College of Physicians had been founded in 1518, the Company of Barber-Surgeons in 1540 and the Society of Apothecaries in 1617. The physicians conducted a perfunctory examination of their candidates, demanding a knowledge of ancient Greek and Latin authors. Yet their members and fellows, who had to be graduates of either Oxford or Cambridge, believed themselves capable of understanding everything medical and advising patients, as well as what they deemed to be their ancillaries, the surgeons and apothecaries, on what should be done in all medical and surgical eventualities.

In 1745 the Company of Surgeons split away from the Barbers, and in 1800 the Company became the Royal College of Surgeons. Neither physicians nor surgeons admitted obstetricians to their number as such, though many surgeons also acted as man-midwives. If a member or fellow of the Royal College of Physicians practised midwifery he was expelled. In 1827 The President of the Royal College, Sir Henry Halford, wrote a letter to the Prime Minister, Sir Robert Peel. He said that the practice of midwifery was 'an act foreign to the habits of gentlemen of enlarged academic education'. In

1834 a surgeon, Sir Anthony Carlisle, told a Select Committee of Parliament enquiring into medical education that 'it is an imposture to pretend that a medical man is required at a labour'. It would seem that midwifery had a long way to go before becoming respectable in the eyes of most members of the medical profession.

There was much general anxiety about the quality and expertise of medical practitioners in the early years of the 19th century. Seventeen Acts were presented to Parliament between 1840 and 1858 all of which tried to bring some order into the training and education of doctors. At last in 1858 the first Medical Act reached the Statute Book. It set up the General Council of Medical Education and Registration of the United Kingdom, as a statutory body, under the Privy Council. The keeping of the Medical Register was the main tool at its disposal. This contained the names of those who had undergone a required education and training in a variety of medical subjects, in prescribed places and for a prescribed period, followed by the passing of an examination, whose content was also prescribed by the Council. The object of the Register and its power resided (and still resides) in the fact that members of the public could examine it to see who was qualified in the fashion laid down by the General Medical Council, and who was not. It did not prohibit the unqualified from practising medicine, nor does it now. When the Register was first compiled it was found that 5,000 out of the 15,000 people practising medicine in England were not qualified by the new standards demanded by the Council. In 1801 the population of the United Kingdom was about 12 million. The figures give some indication of the kind of medical practice then in being.

Women were not admitted to the Register till later. It was thought that if they became doctors they might have to witness unpleasant scenes which would offend their modesty and sensibilities. Midwives and nurses were of course allowed to do so, presumably without shame or affront!

In the original Act there was no mention of midwifery as being part of the necessary training of a medical practitioner. It was not until a further Act of 1886 that the General Medical Council required that at the qualifying examination every doctor must have received a course of instruction and have obtained practical experience in the management of childbirth. The exact words were that a standard of proficiency must have been achieved,

> 'such as sufficiently to guarantee the possession of knowledge and skills requisite for the efficient practice of medicine, surgery and midwifery'.

For midwifery this was an immense step forward, for now it was accepted as a proper discipline for doctors to practise. When midwives called on doctors to help them they could now rely on them having some expertise, however little. But this was an advance on them having no knowledge at all, as must frequently have been the case previously. Before 1886 it had been possible to qualify either as a physician or a surgeon. Thereafter the qualified had to have studied medicine, surgery and midwifery.

Midwives followed a similar path somewhat later. At a meeting of the Obstetrical Society of London in 1858 there were calls by doctors, as there had often been in the past, for the compulsory training of midwives. In 1866 Dr William Farrar of the Statistical Department of the Office of the Registrar General had asked the Society to investigate the causes of infant mortality. The Report found that in villages only 30–90 per cent of births were attended by midwives of any kind. It was worse in small towns, and in larger towns about the same. In some areas of London midwives of any kind were in attendance at only two per cent of births. Further investigation showed that very few midwives had received any instruction and they often showed,

> 'gross ignorance and incompetence, and a complete inability to contend with any difficulty that may occur. In London, on the other hand, it would appear there are many women practising midwifery who have received a certain amount of instruction at various institutions, but these, although fairly competent in the ordinary cases, are also quite unequal to any of the emergencies of obstetrics.'

These criticisms were dire. Little would seem to have changed for centuries. But there were some pioneer women who realized the need for being trained in various hospitals in the metropolis.

In 1870 the Obstetrical Society of London pressed for the compulsory education and formal examination of midwives, to be followed by registration, after the fashion of the doctors. Since this was unlikely to happen quickly the Society established a voluntary examination. Successful candidates were awarded a certificate of the London Obstetrical Society, or LOS. It became much respected and sought after. By the time of the establishment of the first Roll of Midwives in 1902, about one-third of those admitted to it already had the LOS, showing the desire for establishing an incipient profession.

In 1881 a Midwives Institute was founded in London. All its members held the LOS. Its objectives were to raise the standard of midwifery and the status of midwives and to petition Parliament for legislation to control entry to the profession and regulate its practice. The Institute had the support of Florence Nightingale who had earlier arranged with Joseph Lister to have midwives trained at King's College Hospital. She was the moving spirit in properly founding a midwifery school at the General Lying-in Hospital, York Road, after it had been refurbished following its closure on account of puerperal fever deaths. She had as much concern for midwifery as for general nursing. The nursing school she started at St Thomas's Hospital was only a quarter of a mile away from the General Lying-in Hospital. This remained a flagship of training of midwives till its closure in 1971.

As a result of the initiatives of the Midwives Institute a Parliamentary Select Committee was set up in 1892. Their work showed,

> 'that there is at present serious and unnecessary loss of life and health and permanent injury to both mother and child in the treatment of childbirth, and that some legislative provision for improvement and regulation is desirable.'

The result, after some false starts, was the Midwives Act of 1902, which set up the Central Midwives Board. Its development as major force for good came in the 20th century.

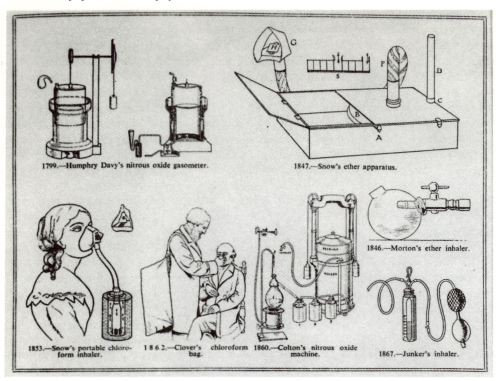

1799.—Humphry Davy's nitrous oxide gasometer.

1847.—Snow's ether apparatus.

1846.—Morton's ether inhaler.

1853.—Snow's portable chloro-form inhaler.

1 8 6 2.—Clover's chloroform bag.

1860.—Colton's nitrous oxide machine.

1867.—Junker's inhaler.

Fig. 9.7: Early use of anaesthetic apparatus

CHAPTER TEN

1900–1950

Introduction

The first half of the 20th century saw most of the problems of labour overcome. This allowed obstetricians and midwives to concentrate on other aspects of the whole childbearing process, notably pregnancy. Antenatal care flourished during this period. This was a significant move in emphasis from crisis management of acute problems to trying to prevent them happening at all, and, if that were not possible, to forestalling their worst consequences. This was especially true of the then so-called toxaemias of pregnancy.

The operations of obstetrics were increasingly successful in their outcomes for both mothers and babies. Pain was virtually controlled or banished by anaesthesia and analgesia. The worst effects of haemorrhages were offset by blood transfusion. Infections were reduced by the practice of antisepsis and asepsis as bacteriological knowledge increased rapidly. Later, infections became curable by chemotherapy and antibiotics.

The ancient grim spectres of obstruction in labour, pain, haemorrhage, infection and fits, all of which had haunted childbearing women for centuries, began to be exorcised. The pace of advance increased year by year. There came a continuity of care throughout pregnancy, labour and the puerperium which had previously not been practised nor thought possible and desirable.

There was change on every front at once. It is therefore difficult to present a continuous narrative of the history of clinical midwifery at this time. The progress was often integrated and not to be neatly unravelled subsequently. Yet it still seems best to attempt to deal with the period under headings similar to those used earlier.

Labour

Abdominal and vaginal palpation in pregnancy and labour helped to define more closely the lie, presentation, position, degree of engagement of the fetal head in the pelvis, and to a lesser extent the size of the fetus. Routine auscultation determined whether the fetus was alive or possibly dead or suffering distress demanding delivery for its survival. These refinements of diagnosis came about gradually and were incorporated into the textbooks without being attributable to individual pioneer obstetricians. The routines of clinical diagnosis became universally accepted.

The lie of the fetus is the relation of its long axis to the long axis of the uterus. It can be longitudinal, oblique or transverse. The presentation can be either the head or the breech in longitudinal or oblique lies. It is usually one or other shoulder or arm in transverse lies.

In the common longitudinal lie the presentation is either of head or breech. With head presentations the head can be well flexed on the trunk, or may be in various degrees of deflexion. When the extension (deflexion) of the head is extreme the face presents over the cervix and brim of the pelvis. Slightly lesser extension results in the brow presenting. In still less extension the top of the head presents. Each of these may bring different problems in labour.

When the breech presents the legs may be fully extended so that the baby's feet are under the chin at the top of the uterus. This is often called a frank breech or a breech with extended legs. In other cases the legs are flexed at the knees and hips so that both the buttocks and feet are over the cervix and brim of the pelvis. These two modes of presentation also may produce special problems in labour.

Position defines the relationship of the fetal head or breech to fixed points on the brim of the bony pelvis. These are the two sacro-iliac joints at the back, and the two ilio-pubic eminences at the front. On the presenting part is what is called the *point of denomination*. This is a defined part of the head or breech. In face presentations it is the chin; in brow presentations the frontal bones; in the well flexed and slightly deflexed head presentations it is the occiput. In any form of breech it is the sacrum.

The classification of these various presentations then becomes left and right occipito-anterior, both of which are well flexed and tend to cause few troubles; left and right occipito-posterior; left and right mento-anterior and mento-posterior (chin); left and right fronto-anterior and fronto-posterior (brow); and left and right sacro-anterior and sacro-posterior in breech presentations. There can be the further addition of transverse positions when the point of denomination on the fetus is midway between a sacro-iliac joint and an ilio-pubic eminence.

Engagement of the head in the pelvic brim is when the widest diameter of the head has settled in the brim or just beyond it, on its journey down the birth canal. It can be determined clinically in most instances by abdominal and vaginal examinations. Its importance lies in the fact that the head is the largest part of the baby. If the head can negotiate the pelvis, then the rest of the body will do so. Moreover in most varieties of small or contracted pelves, especially those due to rickets, the brim is the narrowest part of the bony pelvic canal. If it is sure that the head is engaged then the prognosis for a successful vaginal outcome of labour is usually good.

It has to be realized that obstruction in labour had almost obsessed obstetricians and midwives for centuries. It was the commonest form of difficulty in labour as then understood. The early 20th century began to sort out the different forms of obstruction. Obviously the baby's head can be large or the pelvic canal small and then there is said to be 'disproportion' between the two. But the malpresentations of the deflexed heads may also cause disproportion since as the head extends the diameter as presented to the pelvic brim increases, and this may effectively be a cause of partial or complete obstruction.

The significance of all this variety of presentations and positions and degrees of engagement is that they may call for different schemes of management both prior to and in labour, because of the difficulties they may cause. The realisation of this is due to several unnamed obstetricians and the general diffusion of obstetric ideas through the literature and by conference. It meant that there came to be more clinical precision in diagnosis and accepted means of dealing with the various actual and potential difficulties. Its value at the time can scarcely be overestimated. It became a bedrock of antenatal care and management in labour.

Disproportion and obstruction in labour

In earlier days this was often dealt with by internal version, which, of course, is only possible when labour has progressed quite far. It may be effective for face, brow, and deflexed heads associated with occipito-posterior positions. Unless there is absolute disproportion between the head and the pelvis the head may negotiate the birth canal as the after-coming head of a breech. If disproportion is due to a deflexed head then it may be possible to attempt to flex it manually with a hand in the vagina aided by one on the abdomen. It is an alternative to internal version but is often not successful. In face presentations it may be possible to rotate the whole head by fingers within the pelvis so that the chin comes to the front. It can then be delivered. Even with brow and occipito-posterior presentations the head may manage partially to enter the pelvis and then there is the chance of delivery using forceps, though this may compress the head and delivery may be traumatic for both mother and baby. These methods were tried but were often of no real value.

During the early decades of the century if the baby was dead there was often recourse to perforation of the skull, extracting the brain tissue, breaking up the bones with a cranioclast and extracting the remainder of the head with a cephalotribe. In transverse lie attempts were made to turn the baby, by external version with hands on the abdomen, to either a cephalic or breech presentation in late pregnancy or early labour. Internal or bipolar version to make the breech present was also sometimes possible. If the transverse lie had been neglected in labour then the head had to be severed, in the operation of decapitation, using a Gigli saw to cut through the tissues of the neck.

All these dire interventions were used, early in the century, since caesarean section was still extremely hazardous for the mother. Complications could and did arise from the anaesthetic, from haemorrhage and from sepsis, and often a combination of all three, and all very difficult to deal with using the knowledge and techniques of the time. Every effort was still bent to avoiding its performance. It was a last and dangerous resort.

Uterine action

At this late stage of the development of midwifery there was still much confusion about uterine action, particularly in labour. Braxton Hicks had, of course, in the preceding century described the uterine contractions of pregnancy and how they were continued when the woman went into labour. He believed that although associated with pain in labour the contractions remained essentially of the same nature as those of pregnancy. Subsequent knowledge has confirmed this.

In the early decades of the 20th century it was recognized that the uterus did not always contract efficiently in labour. This, of course, had been known for a long time. The problem was how to define the different forms of inefficiency, and what to do about them. The first classification was into *primary and secondary uterine inertia*. In the first the uterus never seemed to get going at all, contracting feebly without causing much pain. The general tendency in care was to await delivery, however long it took, sometimes several days, provided that there was no maternal or fetal distress. Some doctors attempted to force the uterus to contract more vigorously by giving ergot, as midwives had done for a long time.

In 1909 William Blair Bell (1871–1936) of Liverpool used pituitary extract to increase contractions. It was then a mixture of both the oxytocic factor (causing uterine contractions) and vasopressin (causing contraction of blood vessels). The latter might be dangerous if the woman already had a high blood pressure. It was not until much later that oxytocin was obtained in purer mode and it has come to be widely used in the second half of the century. There is no doubt, however, that Blair Bell was able, through his extract, to make the uterus contract more vigorously when its action was weak. Others, of course, followed the example of Bell in using oxytocin in intravenous drips in primary inertia. The cause of primary inertia was groped for but little came of the speculations, except that there was a general view that it was probably due to maternal anxiety and fear.

Secondary inertia was diagnosed when labour seemed to be progressing more or less normally and then finally came to a stop well before the birth of the baby. It was thought by Braxton Hicks to be due to exhaustion of the muscular powers. Others called it a 'tired uterus'. Because it was tired out it was deemed of no value to attempt to stimulate it with oxytocics of any kind. It dawned on very few at the time that this might be a response to obstruction due to contracted pelvis or malpresentation or malposition.

Truly obstructed labour was thought always to be followed by stormy contractions, great thinning of the lower uterine segment and the formation of a Bandl's retraction ring, with the high possibility of uterine rupture where the upper segment of the uterus meets the lower one.

Then another form of uterine action was called 'colicky'. Such contractions were extremely painful and failed to advance labour. Measurements of the pressure inside the uterus purported to show that it was up to three times the normal of just over 100 mmHg. The condition was thought often to progress to a generally contracted state and possibly to the formation of a constriction ring round the neck of the fetus or less often the abdomen. Clifford White, of London, writing in *Historical Review of British Obstetrics and Gynaecology 1800–1950* described a series of personal cases of constriction ring. He found craniotomy useless, for after this it was still not possible to pull the baby through the ring. Internal version could not be performed. If it were attempted the uterus was ruptured. He had a maternal mortality of 31 per cent with laparotomy, and 58 per cent without it. By 1947 another group had reduced maternal mortality for this condition to nil and fetal mortality to 3.5 per cent in 105 cases.

What seems so odd now is that most modern obstetricians have never seen a case of constriction ring in the first and second stages of labour. Perhaps that is because they rarely put a hand right inside the uterus when the fetus is within it. Constriction rings are only diagnosable by this method, and are possibly caused by it. Moreover if obstetricians meet trouble in a forceps delivery, which they may or may not doubtfully attribute to a constriction ring without positive proof by intrauterine palpation, such that the baby cannot be delivered, then there is now easy resort to caesarean section. This was not so readily the case early in the 20th century because of its very real dangers. Medical efforts to relax a constriction ring were made using amyl nitrite inhaled under an anaesthetic mask. Though constriction ring is now rarely recognized it has to be accepted that it had been written about since Smellie's time, and even before that. It was certainly not a figment of the imagination of older obstetricians. It is simply that the problem is now sidestepped in ways that were not possible earlier.

The only forms of constriction ring now seen are those in the third stage where manual removal of the placenta is needed. The ring can then be definitely present and may be relaxed either by the anaesthetic being given for the operation to be performed, or by inhaled amyl nitrite. The only alternative is to wait until the uterine constriction disappears as it always does in time. It seems probable that constriction rings occur only as a response to intrauterine manipulations.

White, in the same article, recognizes cervical dystocia in which the cervix fails properly to dilate but remains rigid. One author he cites managed to find six varieties of the disorder. This exemplifies the tendency to over-elaborate and play with words when real solutions and comprehension are not available.

The understanding of the clinical varieties of uterine contractions in labour was chaotic until about 1950, when Thomas Norman Arthur Jeffcoate (1907–1993) of Liverpool sorted them out. The scheme was based on clinical observation at the bedside of the strength, frequency and duration of the contractions. Strength was essentially a matter of feeling the hardness of the uterus at the height of a contraction. Frequency was obviously the number of contractions over a given period of time (say ten minutes), and duration was from the time when the contraction appeared to begin to the time when it seemed to fade away. Although these clinical signs lacked precise measurement they were confirmed later to have validity by scientific physiologists and others. Essentially there were:

1. normal contractions;
2. contractions of low intensity using the three observations;
3. contractions of high intensity;
4. irregular contractions (asymmetrical uterine action) – the former colicky uterus;
5. constriction ring;
6. cervical rigidity; and,
7. spurious labour.

The first four of these were most often due to some degree of obstruction due to contracted pelvis, malpresentation or malposition. If these could be dealt with then it was probable that the uterus would resume normal contractions. If such a cause could be corrected or eliminated from further consideration, then normal contractions could probably be restored by the use of a pitocin (oxytocin) drip, perhaps after priming the patient with oestrogen. This brilliant piece of clinical work stripped away most of the former delusions, and offered methods of diagnosis and treatment. It was a breath of fresh air in a previously obscure and befogged situation. Rationality had been imported. It transformed understanding and management.

Spurious labour was recognized by failure of the contractions to increase in strength, frequency and duration, over time, and failure of the cervix to dilate. It was essential to recognize the condition and treat it by sedation and analgesia, since otherwise the woman thought she had been in labour for a long time, when in fact she was not. Her attendants might be misled as well, becoming unnecessarily anxious and perhaps persuading themselves to detrimental interference of some kind. The dividing line between uncomfortable Braxton Hicks contractions of pregnancy and the painful contractions of true advancing labour is very imprecise.

The various forms of abnormal uterine action often caused maternal distress or fetal distress or both and also delay in delivery. These all demand careful monitoring in labour, as well as looking out for the nature of the uterine action so that decisions can be made as to when to intervene and in what manner, if at all. Maternal distress was recognized as being both psychological and physical in the middle years of the century. Physical signs were those of anxiety, pain, raised pulse and blood pressure, and diminished output of urine. Fetal distress was diagnosed by a slow or rapid fetal heart rate – below 120 or above 160 beats per minute, and slow return to a normal rate. This, of course, was then counted clinically through a fetal stethoscope on the abdomen. In cephalic presentations there might also be the passage of meconium from the fetal bowel. Delay in the first stage of labour was diagnosed by delay in the dilatation of the cervix and the overall length of true labour. It was then accepted that a normal labour could last for 24 hours or even more. The second stage of labour was often of two hours and the third stage of one hour.

It will be seen that there were slow changes in understanding and management of many aspects of labour, including those of uterine contractions and their variations. So many of the problems became soluble by the increasing safety of caesarean section, forceps and breech delivery, anaesthesia, blood transfusion and efficacious prevention and treatment of infection.

Obstetric operations

External version

This operation of turning the fetus within the uterus by purely abdominal manipulations and usually from breech to cephalic presentation was introduced by J.H. Wigand (1769–1817) in 1807, but was not used much generally until the 20th century. This was probably due to the growth of antenatal care and the awareness of the dangers to the fetus of breech delivery. Older obstetricians had no fears of breech delivery, and often welcomed it. The fetal mortality was often well over ten per cent. Making the head rather than the breech present seemed to be good preventative care, except to those still addicted to internal version and breech extraction as a way out of most difficulties.

Keith Vartan, of the London Hospital, in 1945 showed that spontaneous version from breech to head rarely occurred after 33 weeks of pregnancy. There was then a relatively large amount of liquor relative to the fetus. Version was therefore usually performed at about 34 weeks, when it often seemed to be successful. It was almost always successful in transverse lies, for they occur in multigravidae with lax abdominal walls and uterus and a large amount of liquor amnii. It was always worthwhile to prevent a woman going into labour with a transverse lie because of its possibly dire complications. Later, some doubt was thrown on the notion that external cephalic version really reduced the overall numbers of breech deliveries. Nevertheless it was always worth a try if it could be done without great force. There were some who would follow failed version by external version under anaesthesia. It had some merit when the patient was anxious and tense and thus firmly contracted her abdominal muscles, making version difficult. However, this was quickly abandoned because excessive force could be used and might separate the placenta from its bed, and there was always the possible complication of entangling the cord round some part of the fetus, and so obstructing its circulation. Nevertheless without anaesthesia the operation was widely performed.

Induction of labour

Attempts to induce the onset of labour are of great antiquity. In the 18th century Thomas Denman of the Middlesex Hospital used it in order to prevent the baby growing too big and perhaps then liable to obstruct labour. It did not have much vogue, no doubt because it often failed. The usual method was to stretch the cervix manually near term and perhaps rupture the membranes with a finger nail or scissors. An enema too was often given. Of course the method is sometimes successful, but by no means always.

Krause had added to this method the insertion of stiff bougies between the membranes and the lower uterine segment. Others, such as Champetier de Ribes, had used fluid-filled bags to lie within the lower uterine segment and distend it. All these methods were unreliable. They were known as surgical inductions.

In 1920 B.P. Watson of New York advocated medical induction, using castor oil and quinine. Castor oil was known to cause contraction of the colon and rectum and by a sort of sympathetic action it might cause the uterus to contract too. An enema was given prior to this dose. Quinine came to be used since it had been observed that pregnant patients given the drug for malaria often went into labour. This apparently innocuous method was used worldwide, the quinine being given in high enough doses to cause ringing in the ears (tinnitus) – a toxic side-effect. It is doubtful if the method was really efficacious. But it had the merit of staying the hand of the obstetrician from invading the vagina and opening up the amniotic cavity. This is certain to introduce infection if the onset of labour is delayed by more than about 24 hours. Both mother and baby may then be infected and be caused to have a serious illness, perhaps even leading to death. Bougies and bags were even more likely to introduce infection than other methods.

In an attempt to reduce the possibility of infection Drew Smythe of Bristol in 1937 devised a double curved metal catheter. This was in theory slipped through the cervix and round the head of the fetus so that its point (with a removable stylet) pierced only the hindwaters above the head. A reasonable amount of fluid was then withdrawn so making the uterus contract as its volume diminished. It often failed. The instrument might puncture the forewaters lying over the cervix and sometimes it would catch and lift up an edge of the placenta, if it were low-lying and posterior. Bleeding, occasionally severe, could be caused.

Getting a woman to go into labour for certain at a predetermined time was still a largely unsolved problem during the whole of the first half of the 20th century, despite a variety of manipulative 'surgical' efforts and drugs of little proven value.

Forceps

Forceps became a routine part of midwifery practice during the first half of the 20th century, largely because of the use of general anaesthesia. Their use had been codified and the indications and conditions for application were universally accepted over time. The commonest type of forceps was that introduced by James Young Simpson, but there were many others, of similar pattern, such as those of Neville-Barnes and Milne Murray. Several had axis traction rods or handles with a view to being able to exert the pull on the fetal head in conformity with the curve of Carus. They were really only necessary where the head was not fully engaged in the pelvic brim, i.e. the old 'high head'. This operation can be so traumatic to both fetus and mother that it was slowly abandoned in favour of caesarean section. This had become much less hazardous than heretofore. The essential indications for forceps delivery (only in the second stage with the cervix fully dilated) were:

1.   maternal distress;
2.   fetal distress; and,
3.   delay in the second stage.

Maternal distress was obvious enough on psychological and physical grounds. Fetal distress was diagnosed by auscultation of the heart and counting the rate. The normal rate was about 120 beats per minute. It slowed during contractions but then rapidly recovered. If the beats were persistently below 120 per minute or if there was slow recovery to the normal rate after a contraction then fetal distress was certain. A persistent rate of up to 160 beats per minute was also a sure sign of distress. The passage of meconium was an additional sign if the head presented.

Delay in the second stage was diagnosed in the early part of the century when there was no advance of the head over the course of two hours. It was properly reduced to one hour later on. The conditions for the application of the forceps were established and accepted. They were:

1.   the bladder must be empty;
2.   the head must be engaged;
3.   the membranes must be ruptured;
4.   the cervix must be fully dilated;
5.   the occiput must be anterior;
6.   there must be a reasonable chance of delivery through the bony pelvis without force.

The bladder had to be empty to avoid damage to it. The head had to be engaged so that no attempt should be made to deliver a high head. The likely cause of that would be contracted pelvis or brow presentation. The membranes had to be ruptured because if the forceps are applied outside them the blades slip off. The cervix had to be fully dilated to avoid tearing it. In cephalic presentations which were flexed the occiput had to be brought to the front of the pelvis, usually by the use of the four fingers of one hand, to produce an occipito-anterior presentation.

Occasionally the forceps were used when the occiput was posterior and the head well down in the pelvis and when it was impossible to rotate it to the front. Also, in face presentation when the chin is anterior, delivery with the forceps is possible without attempting to change the presentation, though it may be necessary manually to rotate the head so that the chin is made to be anterior.

Manual rotation of the head within the pelvis can be difficult. The whole hand cannot be used for, if it should be, the head has to be pushed up above the pelvic brim, and forceps application should not then be attempted. In manual rotation, therefore, the thumb has to remain outside the vulva. The four fingers have to seek some sort of purchase on the slippery wet head, sometimes using just friction and sometimes the groove behind the fetal ear or a skull suture. Attempts were sometimes made to rotate the head using the forceps in the Scanzoni manoeuvre, but the usual forceps have a pelvic curve on them which if used carelessly describe a wide arc within the vagina and may tear it extensively and also the deeper tissues.

Then came the brilliant new type of forceps from Caspar Gabriel Kielland (1871–1941) of Oslo, in 1915. These had only the slightest pelvic curve and so, whatever the position of the head within the pelvis, they could be applied to it properly over the ears. The other innovation was that the lock, where the handles cross one another, was not fixed but sliding. If the head were tilted to one or other shoulder (asynclitism) then still the blades could be applied to fit on to the baby's head perfectly. As the extraction of the baby commenced the asynclitism was corrected, by the two halves of the forceps sliding upon one another. But even better was the fact that the shanks between the handles and the blades were rounded so that they caused little trauma to the area of the urethra under the symphysis pubis.

Kiellands' method of application was to push the anterior blade up into the cavity of the uterus with the cephalic curve pointing towards the abdominal wall. It was then rotated within the cavity and pulled down to settle on to the baby's head. This was later abandoned in favour of inserting the first blade laterally in the pelvis, then sliding it round the head to fit properly over the anterior ear. With the blades on the head the forceps could be eased up and down a little while gentle rotation was attempted until the right place for this to occur was found.

Rotating the head was usually surprisingly easy. Pulling the head out of the birth canal was, however, more difficult because the handles had been deliberately set backwards from, yet parallel to, the blades. They pressed hard on the perineum, so that a large episiotomy was needed to avoid serious tearing. Because of this many obstetricians took the Kiellands forceps off the head, after rotation, and applied the more usual variety for extraction. The Kiellands forceps were so appropriate for the task of rotating the head within the pelvis that they became used worldwide, and especially in Europe. The commonest indication for their use was in the occipito-transverse positions when the head stuck transversely, in so-called 'deep transverse arrest', and would not rotate one way or the other in the pelvis. But the Kielland forceps could be used for rotation whatever the position of the head within the pelvis.

An excellent different type of forceps for dealing with deep transverse arrest was first used in 1924 by Lyman Guy Barton (1866–1944) of Essex County, New York, who invented the instrument. It had a fixed very curved blade which fitted into the hollow of the sacrum, and over one or other of the baby's ears. The other blade was hinged and was slipped over the ear under the symphysis pubis. When in place rotation of the head was easily accomplished and then other forceps were used to deliver it.

In 1936 Arthur Joseph Wrigley (1902–1984) of St Thomas's Hospital, London, produced very light small forceps. They had normal light pelvic and cephalic curves, but the handles were reduced to about 2–3". Apart from the pelvic curve they were very similar to the straight forceps used by William Smellie. The reason for these new forceps was to try to make domiciliary delivery by relatively inexperienced general practitioners safe. At the time nearly all deliveries took place in homes or nursing homes. Wrigley's forceps could only be used when the head was very low in the pelvis, almost at the outlet. Because of the small handles very little compression could be exerted on the head. It was virtually impossible to use two hands for traction so this had to be gently done using one hand only. They made doctors comply with the conditions for the application of the forceps whether they formally knew them or not. They also became very useful in the extraction of the after-coming head of the breech. This was also neatly dealt with by special forceps designed in 1929 by Edmund Brown Piper (1881–1935) of Philadelphia.

Episiotomy

This surgical cutting of the pelvic floor was almost too frequently used during this 50 years. In normal deliveries when the perineum seemed likely to tear it was cut, usually with scissors, the cut being directed away from the anal margin. It was often done by both midwives and doctors without any form of anaesthesia. It was timed to be at the height of a painful contraction on the assumption that it would not then be felt. However the operation did and does have useful purposes in removing obstruction to the head or breech in the last minutes of the second stage, and in preventing tears into the anal sphincter and rectum. If such a tear is inadequately repaired the result may be faecal incontinence. If an episiotomy does not heal well, at least the woman was spared the fistula. Fortunately more recent advances have shown improvement for mothers recovering from this apparently minor operation, which can have such dire consequences in pain and dyspareunia. It is horrifying to recall too that in these 50 years the repair of episiotomies and tears was frequently performed without anaesthesia of any kind.

With most forceps deliveries, except the simplest, it was often necessary to perform an episiotomy. But forceps deliveries were carried out under general anaesthesia and the repair was performed before the anaesthesia was ended.

Internal version

This operation had been used for centuries to overcome problems in labour. It was still used in the period under consideration by many of the older obstetricians. It was of course not only valueless in cases of disproportion but downright dangerous, yet a few still used it for that. If the head will not come through the brim when the head presents it will not come either when it is coming after the body.

The main value of internal version was in transverse lies, and in the delivery of the second twin when the head was not engaged. In experienced hands it might have been useful at a time when caesarean section was never to be lightly entered upon. The operation of internal version was also much used by older obstetricians for relatively minor degrees of placenta praevia, where a hand could be inserted into the uterine cavity beyond the placenta. With a leg brought down it was possible to pull on it or even attach a light weight to it by a bandage so that pressure was exerted on the bleeding placental site. It was called 'plugging with the half-breech'. The days of the operation were numbered as caesarean section became safer and domiciliary practice greatly diminished.

Destructive operations

When forceps delivery failed or there was a high head with the baby dead it was still not uncommon in the first quarter of the century to perform perforation of the head, break up its bones with a cranioclast and extract the remains with a cephalotribe. They were a usual part of the instrumental armamentarium of all labour wards. A Gigli saw was also needed for decapitation of the fetus in neglected transverse lies, with the baby dead. Time has fortunately left these terrible instruments in the museum, never to be used again.

Breech delivery

Nearly always breech deliveries were conducted without thought of the alternative of caesarean section. This was only considered when the bony pelvis was manifestly very small on clinical examination, or when its radiological measurements showed it to be greatly contracted. The technique of delivery was standardized.

In flexed breech a foot was hooked out with the fingers as soon as it was seen at the vulva. When the shoulders appeared an arm was hooked out too. The fetal back was rotated to the front of the mother. A finger was placed in the mouth and delivery was effected with jaw-flexion-shoulder-traction in the so-called Mauriceau-Smellie-Veit manoeuvre.

With extended legs it was usual to wait until the breech emerged from the vulva and the backs of the knees could be seen. When pressed on in the popliteal fossae the legs would flex and a foot could then be easily reached and pulled out as before. Sometimes extended arms would hold up delivery. By running two fingers over the shoulder and down the upper arm to sweep the whole arm across the chest it was brought down, and the procedure could be repeated on the other side. The head could then be delivered by forceps, perhaps Piper's, sliding the blades along the underside of the body to be applied along a correct line running from the chin to the vertex.

Breech extraction was sometimes called for when there was fetal distress, maternal distress or serious delay, and time was deemed to be short for the baby. The patient was given a general anaesthetic, legs were brought down, or traction exerted in the groin, followed by traction on the pelvis and body, the arms were brought down and the head delivered with forceps.

Regrettably all these manoeuvres might cause injury to the baby. A humerus might be fractured. So might a femur. Rather worse was when traction on the arms might cause Erb's paralysis or Klumpke's paralysis. The first was due to traction on the upper parts of the brachial plexus leading to various forms of paralysis of the arm. Klumpke's paralysis was due to traction on the lower cords of the plexus and led to paralysis in the hand and forearm regions. The rapidity with which the head sometimes had to be delivered could cause intracranial haemorrhage, leading to mental retardation among other things. Wilhelm Heinrich Erb (1840–1921) described his palsy in 1873, though it had been noted by Smellie much earlier.

Despite the tendency to persist with vaginal delivery in breech presentation the overall results for the baby were not good. As late as 1949 Robert Newton of St Mary's Hospital, Manchester, found that over the previous 12 years the fetal mortality there was 7.1 per cent. Earlier in the century it might very well have been worse. Yet there is almost no maternal mortality with a breech vaginal delivery, while that for caesarean section could perhaps have seemed prohibitive to older obstetricians.

Caesarean section

This became increasingly used. It was essentially the classical operation in which the abdominal incision is about 6" long and beginning slightly above and to the right of the navel. Going between the two rectus muscles and through the peritoneum the uterus is easily reached and incised until the baby and the placenta can be delivered. With anaesthesia it must be one of the easiest operations anatomically in the book. But the haemorrhage from the cut uterus can be terrifying. In the early years there was little or no availability of blood transfusion, and there was the ever present danger of infection, which was not always preventable, and when it did take hold there were no specific remedies for it.

In England for cases of contracted pelvis Eardley Holland (1879–1967) of London and Munro Kerr (1868–1960) of Glasgow found the maternal mortality from caesarean section for the years from 1911 to 1920 was just under two per cent when the patient was not in labour. But it rose to ten per cent if the operation was late in labour, 14 per cent if surgical induction had been performed, and to a shocking 27 per cent if attempts had been made to effect vaginal delivery before the abdominal section. The causes were surgical shock, haemorrhage and infection. Even fetal mortality was high at five per cent in the simpler cases, at 16 per cent late in labour and 37 per cent after attempts at vaginal delivery. There can be no wonder that all were chary of undertaking the operation except upon the most compelling indications, when no other choice was left.

Trial or test of labour

In the fourth decade of the century when caesarean section had become safer because of better anaesthesia, blood transfusion and the start of chemotherapy, there came the concept of the 'trial of labour'. This was conducted when there seemed clinical or radiological doubts about the capacity of the pelvis to allow the fetal head safely through it. This might be due to contracted pelvis or large head giving rise to disproportion. It was by no means easy to determine whether there was disproportion in any given case. Moreover the strength of uterine contractions could not be foretold.

The trial of labour really meant the very close monitoring of progress in the first stage. It meant assessment of maternal fortitude and any psychological or physical distress. The latter was measured by pulse rate, blood pressure, temperature and fluid balance. The strength, frequency and duration of uterine contractions were observed. The fetus was monitored by its heart rate, looking for any signs of distress. The progress of labour was observed for descent of the head as determined by abdominal and vaginal examinations. The head was examined vaginally for signs of compression by moulding and by the caput succedaneum (the boggy oedematous lump raised on the scalp when there is head compression). Also important was the rate of dilatation of the cervix. With such a series of observations it was usually possible to decide whether the labour should go on or whether it should be terminated for the benefit of one or other patient, or both, by caesarean section.

There was still much anxiety about contracted pelvis and disproportion. Trial of labour was a valuable way of dealing with it, leaving sensible decision about the method of delivery as late as possible. Many women subjected to this method delivered quite normally. It was only in the second half of the century that it was recognized that what will happen in any labour cannot be forecast. Now every labour has become a 'trial' in the professional sense. There is close monitoring of all the factors of labour, with better recording than there used to be.

Obstetric radiology

X-rays were discovered in 1895 by Wilhelm Conrad Röntgen (1845–1923). As early as 1896 H. Varnier of France had produced a radiograph of a fetus within the excised uterus from a woman recently dead. There were immense problems in getting unblurred pictures of the live moving fetus in pregnancy. Rays scattered widely giving a fuzzy negative. Exposures had to be very long, lasting minutes. In 1903 Heinrich Ernst Albers-Schönberg (1865–1921) invented a compression diaphragm which minimized the scattering. In 1913 Gustav Bucky (1880–1963) and Hollis Elmer Potter (b.1880) used moving grids to prevent scatter. X-ray machines increased in power. Films were made more sensitive. Short exposure times became possible so that blurring due to fetal movement was eliminated.

With X-rays the fetal skeleton could be seen in utero from about 16 weeks onwards, giving absolute proof of pregnancy, obtainable in no other way. Late in pregnancy the lie, presentation and position of the fetus could be diagnosed for sure. Multiple pregnancy could be confirmed with certainty. Abnormalities such as hydrocephalus, spina bifida and anencephaly could be demonstrated. Death of the fetus was shown by Spalding's sign. When the baby has been dead for some time the brain shrinks and the skull bones then overlap at the sutures. A.B. Spalding (1874–1942) of the USA first described this in 1922.

It can be of importance to estimate the maturity of the fetus especially near term. Postmaturity and prematurity are both preferably avoided. Radiology can show the presence of a secondary epiphyseal ossification centre in the lower end of the femur at about 36 weeks and in the upper end of the tibia at about 40 weeks. Other bones, particularly of the foot also have fairly definite times of appearance of ossification centres. This technique was widely used.

In a few cases of breech presentation it was sometimes possible to measure the biparietal diameter of the head, when conditions were favourable. This allowed comparison with the size of the pelvis and gave an indication of the safety of breech delivery with the after-coming head. This measurement was first accomplished in 1935 by L.N. Reece.

As a result of the obsessive anxiety of obstetricians over the centuries with contracted pelves and disproportion the really major advance seemed to them to be the definite measurements of the diameters of the pelvis. With varying positions of the woman, and careful positioning of the X-ray tube and the film, and some mathematical calculation, it became possible to measure all pelvic diameters as well as the shape of the brim, cavity and outlet, assess pelvic tilt and the lumbo-sacral angle and the subpubic arch. It seemed as if a new era had dawned.

Herbert Thoms (1885–1972) and William Edgar Caldwell (1880–1943) working with Howard Carman Moloy (1903–1953) in the USA produced a series of papers around 1930. Often they used stereoscopic methods to give three dimensional representations of the bony pelvis. They identified four parent types which they named gynaecoid, android, anthropoid and platypelloid. The first was the normal female pelvis of average size with rounded brim, cavity and outlet, with a subpubic arch of about a right angle. The android pelvis was male-like with conventional stylised heart-shaped brim, narrow at the front. The cavity and the outlet tended to be smaller than the brim, and the subpubic arch narrow. The anthropoid pelvis was ape-like, in that it was oval at the brim, its long axis being from front to back, and that same shape persisted in the cavity and outlet. The platypelloid pelvis was broad from side to side.

Apart from the gynaecoid pelvis each shape was associated with a variety of difficulties in delivery. There might be non-engagement of the head, or failure to descend through a funnel pelvis. There could be malpositions and malpresentations. With measurements of these pelves it was a question of being forewarned and so forearmed to deal with potential problems.

A well-recognized pelvis was that due to rickets, with its distorted brim shape, protrusions into the cavity by the femoral heads, tilting backwards of the sacrum, which could sometimes be convex rather than concave. There were similar distortions in osteomalacia of older malnourished women. The rachitic pelvis is undoubtedly due to lack of vitamin D in childhood. It began to be suspected that the other varieties of pelvis might be due to subclinical rickets, especially in the android type. This theory is probably true and the variant shapes may be due to malnutrition rather than being of genetic origin. There is some evidence too that the anthropoid pelvis is commoner in well-nourished women.

Radiologists, because of their precise measurements of both head and pelvis, began to offer prognoses for labour. Obstetricians went along with them for there came a vogue for having a full X-ray pelvimetry on every primigravida, so that everything about her bony pelvis could be known. There were sometimes radiological reports suggesting that forceps delivery or caesarean section would be needed. These ignored the fact that the progress of labour is not simply a mechanical matter of getting the fetus through a bony ring. Especially uterine action and maternal and fetal reaction to labour cannot be assessed before labour. It was partly this ignorant mechanical attitude that led to the introduction of the 'trial of labour', the technique of which has been described.

There were many inductions of labour to offset the perceived evils of disproportion because of these pelvic measurements. But doubts about this crept in. Arthur Joseph Wrigley of St Thomas's Hospital in 1934 analysed the results of this policy in five London hospitals. Judging by the absence of moulding of the head due to compression he found that about 50 per cent of the inductions had probably been unnecessary and perhaps harmful.

Later still in the second half of the century it was realized that the excessive radiation involved in a full X-ray pelvimetry was dangerous for the fetus in particular. The excessive use of radiology which characterized the 1940s and 1950s was fortunately then reduced and its proper indications established. There is always a tendency to overuse new techniques when they are first introduced. As time passes the drawbacks are learned, and proper indications gradually emerge.

Obstetric radiology obviously became a most valuable diagnostic tool for the reasons enumerated. That it was used excessively was no fault of the method, but rather of enthusiastic users of it, who wished to make childbirth ever safer. They did not at first realise the several drawbacks of the technique.

Relief of pain

There were few serious attempts to relieve the pain of labour until the time of James Young Simpson. Thereafter the usual anaesthetics were nitrous oxide, ether and chloroform. Other drugs such as chloral hydrate were tried in other fields, but were not imported into midwifery. Local anaesthesia with novocaine (later called procaine) was written about in 1905 in a book by Friedrich Wilhelm Braun (1862–1934) of Leipzig. But it was not at first used in midwifery. The administration of local anaesthetics and intravenous therapy were made possible by the introduction into Europe of the hypodermic hollow needle and syringe by Francis Rynd (1803–1861) of Dublin in 1845.

Chloroform and ether were used by dripping them, originally on to a handkerchief or cloth, but later there were metal masks covered with lint. It was well described as 'rag and bottle'. An inhaler, devised by Ferdinand Ethelbert Junker (1828–1901) in 1867 was often used for chloroform. The anaesthetic was put in a bottle and by a hand bulb pumping air it was vaporized to reach an ill-fitting mask over the face. This allowed excess of the drug to escape. An anaesthetic in vogue for major surgery was a mixture of two parts chloroform to three parts of ether.

For most operations, such as forceps, breech extraction, manual removal of placenta and caesarean section, administration of general anaesthesia came to be by using Boyle's machine. Henry Edmund Gaskin Boyle (1875–1941) had devised this during the war of 1914–18. Metered nitrous oxide and oxygen were blown over drugs such as ether, which was carried into the lungs with the gases. A better anaesthetic gas for obstetrics was cyclopropane used in surgery in 1934 by John A. Stiles and others. It was much used in obstetrics about 1950. Chloroform had been ousted from the anaesthetic armamentarium because it could cause gross liver damage and even death. Slowly ether disappeared too as better and safer drugs were produced, which especially caused less respiratory depression in the newborn.

Pentothal, now thiopentone, was introduced into surgical practice for induction of anaesthesia in 1935. It came into use later in obstetrics. It was much better than the prior method which had the patient breathing nitrous oxide gas directly from the mask until she was nearly unconscious. It was a most unpleasant and often terrifying experience. Pentothal needed only a small amount injected into a vein and the patient lost consciousness almost immediately, and the anaesthetic could then be switched to a gaseous one. Relaxants of muscle are an invaluable aid for the surgeon. They allow easier access to the part to be operated on and less anaesthesia may be needed. Curare was the first of the relaxants introduced in 1942. Flaxedil (gallamine triethiodide) came in 1946.

These general anaesthetics were not really suitable for controlling the pain of early labour, for this may go on for some hours. A valuable approach to this problem was made by Carl Joseph Gauss (1875–1957) of Freiburg. It was called 'twilight sleep', and was first used in 1902. It consisted of regularly repeated intramuscular doses of morphine and scopolamine (hyoscine), starting early in labour and carried on throughout it. Gauss's book was called *Geburten in Künstliche Dammerschlaf* (Birth with induced clouded consciousness). He reported on 500 cases saying,

> 'The *Dammerschlaf* produced by scopolamine-morphine is able to limit the suffering of the woman in labour to the lowest minimum imaginable. This objective is attained without disagreeable secondary effects upon the subjective condition of the woman in labour, without substantial interference with the labour itself, without danger to the mother, without injury to the child.'

Not only was there good relief of pain but there was also forgetting (amnesia) of many of the subjective events of labour. To many midwives and obstetricians this seemed to be especially valuable. Unfortunately by pushing the doses of the drugs to their limit some women were made delirious and many babies suffered respiratory depression at birth due to the morphine.

Despite the drawbacks it was a serious attempt to deal with a previously neglected problem of childbirth. It seemed to be a great boon to many women and their midwifery assistants, and was widely used throughout the world, especially in the 1920s and 1930s, despite the often deleterious effects on the baby. For a very long time mothers were deemed to be more important than their new babies. It was only when midwifery became very much safer for mothers that attention slowly swung to better care of the baby, both before and after birth. It was a gradual process of changing attitudes both by health professionals and the laity.

'Twilight sleep' was less used after the introduction of pethidine (dolantin) in 1939 by O. Eisler and O. Schaumann in Germany. It caused much less respiratory depression in the newborn than morphine. The scopolamine was dropped, usually in favour of a barbiturate. The first of these – barbital – had been synthesized in 1902. Many others followed and Evipan came in 1932 and was much used. Barbiturates were intended to diminish the anxiety of labour and so perhaps help to reduce the pain felt. The drawbacks of these drugs were only slowly realized. They can, by affecting the fetal liver, lower the vitamin K in the baby and so lead to neonatal bleeding. Nevertheless for a long time in the 1940s and just after the usual procedure was to use both barbiturates and pethidine, the last often repeated frequently to ease the pain of the first stage of labour. Nitrous oxide and air, or preferably oxygen helped with the pain experienced just before full dilatation of the cervix and during the second stage.

Sporadic attempts were made to introduce spinal anaesthesia into midwifery practice. Astonishingly the first successful anaesthetic of this kind for a surgical operation was administered by James Leonard Corning (1855–1923) of New York as early as 1885. He used cocaine. By 1902 Fernand Cathelin (b.1873) of Paris used caudal anaesthesia. In this the needle is inserted into the hiatus at the lower end of the sacrum. Under pressure the drug is forced up the spinal canal outside the dura mater, in the epidural space. There it is not in direct contact with the spinal cord, which can be easily damaged beyond repair by some drugs and their contaminants in full spinal anaesthesia. In the epidural space the anaesthetic surrounds the sacral and lumbar nerves, encased in sleeves of dura mater, which transmit painful impulses from the uterus, cervix and vagina. Caudal anaesthesia was much used, with a variety of agents, about 1950 by obstetricians rather than anaesthetists. These specialists came rather late to pain relief in obstetrics.

Local anaesthesia, by procaine (novocaine), in obstetric practice was introduced in 1927 by G. Gellhorn. It was essentially an infiltration of the subcutaneous tissues, muscles and subvaginal tissues of the perineum. It was often used for easing the pain of the last stage of delivery of the fetal head, and also for the performance of episiotomy and its repair. About the mid-century the more precise technique of pudendal nerve block was introduced. A long flexible needle, attached to a syringe of anaesthetic, was passed either through the perineum or the vagina to reach the ischial spines, where the pudendal nerve is close to the bone. It was valuable for low forceps delivery, where the head needed simple lifting out of the birth canal.

In 1933 Robert James Minnitt (1889–1974) introduced his gas (nitrous oxide) and air machine for self administration by women in labour. The principle was essentially better than the use of injected drugs at the end of the first stage, since gases are so rapidly inhaled and exhaled. Nitrous oxide from cylinders ran through a tube to a face mask which the woman held herself. A simple valve allowed the gas to reach her nose and mouth when she drew in a deep breath. But this could only be inhaled when she closed a hole near the face mask with a finger. When she became drowsy her finger fell off the hole and the mask fell away from her face, giving her time to recover before the next pain occurred. It was brilliant in conception and had wide acceptance. It was so safe that by 1936 the Royal College of Obstetricians and Gynaecologists recommended that gas and air could be used by midwives on their own in domiciliary and other practice. It became a common sight to see a midwife driving up to a house in a Morris Minor and then get out of it complete with her bag and a case containing nitrous oxide cylinders and the simple anaesthetic apparatus.

Although often bringing great comfort the gas and air was not always fully efficacious in the relief of pain. The machine was designed to deliver 50 per cent gas and 50 per cent air. Since air consists of 20 per cent oxygen, the woman breathed in only ten per cent of this vital gas. This could render her anoxic, and this may have been the cause of much of the analgesia. But for its time the apparatus was valuable.

There followed the use of 'Trilene' or trichlorethylene. It was known as a cleaning fluid, but was first used as an anaesthetic in 1935. Freedman in 1943 devised a system for its self administration in labour, on the same principles as the Minnitt apparatus. But the great advantage was that the container for 'Trilene' was light whereas gas cylinders were heavy. Moreover 'Trilene' is much more effective as an analgesic. By 1955 the Royal College of Obstetricians and Gynaecologists felt that 'Trilene' in a modified Freedman inhaler was safe for use by midwives practising on their own, provided they had been trained to use it.

Both 'Trilene' and gas and air were immensely valuable because they were widely available through midwives to large numbers of women wherever they might be in labour, home, nursing home or hospital. Before this the only way to relieve them had been by continued interrupted administration of ether or chloroform, which over a long period was dangerous to both mother and baby and required the presence of a doctor to give the drugs.

A quite new approach to controlling the feelings of pain in labour came with the work of Grantly Dick Read (1890–1959) of London, when he published his *Natural Childbirth* in 1933. He followed this with *Childbirth without Fear* in 1942. His thesis was that most of the pain of childbirth was due to fear, anxiety and apprehension. Fear caused muscular tension which in its turn caused pain. He called this the Fear-Tension-Pain Syndrome. He coined the aphorism 'tense woman, tense cervix'. Tension in the cervix and its resistance to the action of the muscular contractions of the body of the uterus was, in his thought, a major cause of excessive pain in labour. The way to diminish tension was for the woman to:

1.   learn about the processes of all phases of childbirth, so that they would be understood and not feared;
2.   learn how to relax when under stress so that general muscular tension was reduced to a minimum;
3.   control breathing as an aid to overcoming tension.

There was therefore emphasis on educational antenatal classes and relaxation and breathing exercises under the tuition of physiotherapists and midwives. Later, much of this teaching was undertaken by lay women, often under the auspices of the Natural Childbirth Trust. During labour the woman was also never to be left alone to cope with her problems for herself. Again to diminish fear the woman was to be taken, when pregnant, to see the labour wards where she would be delivered so that she had some idea of what to expect. The reasons for the variety of apparatus had to be explained to her.

The theory on which all this was based was, to say the least, suspect. But that it had, and still has, enormously beneficial effects for some women is sure. For the first time there was formal recognition of the importance of psychology in all the processes of childbirth. Of course, this fact was dimly perceived by a great many midwives and obstetricians, but all they tended to do was attempt to give reassurance and kind words. Now they were being shown that it was possible to do much more than this. Despite the criticisms the system often worked in practice, so it scarcely mattered if the theory was sound or unsound. There was certainty of interaction of psychological and physical factors.

Natural childbirth was enthusiastically received by many women, not surprisingly. But unfortunately many of them came to expect painless childbirth as a result of their own efforts. Dick Read never offered this, though some women really did not experience much pain. He never eschewed the use of pain-killing drugs if and when these were needed, and preferably at the request of the woman herself. His objective was to remove fear, as far as that was possible. He knew he could not always relieve pain through the relaxation and breathing methods he advocated so well. The result sometimes was that some women felt that they were failures if they did not have a painless labour, and even greater failures if events dictated that they had to have a forceps or abdominal delivery. They felt they had let themselves, their husbands and families down. Or they blamed those who had taught them or attended them. The psychological results could be very distressing for all concerned. The other valid criticism was that the methods tended to be adopted and applied only by better educated women. In this sense it could not therefore be as universally applied as might have been wished. Poorer working women, often with families, were not always able to find the time to attend the antenatal classes.

Yet there can be no doubt that 'natural childbirth' added a new dimension of thought about childbirth and its significance for women and their husbands and families. Husbands were asked to attend the antenatal classes and assist their wives with the techniques of relaxation and breathing. They were encouraged to accompany their wives and help them during labour in all three stages. Also 'natural childbirth' heightened awareness of these formerly unperceived problems by midwives, doctors and ancillary health workers, so that attitudes to childbearing gradually changed for the better. The emotions were seen to be of supreme importance in all aspects of reproduction. 'Natural childbirth' highlighted them and showed that they were worth formal study and appreciation.

Obstetricians themselves often used to use 'rag and bottle' general anaesthesia throughout much of this period. Of course they used local anaesthesia too, mainly as an infiltration of the perineum, and they administered caudal anaesthesia. But as more and more drugs and esoteric techniques of anaesthesia were developed it became obvious that specialists were needed to use them. At first anaesthetists were generalists in their subject, though inevitably there had to come specialization in anaesthesia for neurosurgery, cardiac and chest surgery, and ultimately it was recognized that obstetric anaesthesia had its special needs, so that anaesthetists gradually developed the means required for greater safety of both mother and baby. As they were skilled in resuscitation too they came to play a major part in the immediate care of the newborn, especially in the establishment of respiration.

By the 1950s pain in childbirth could be largely controlled by a variety of means. The ancient curse of Eve had to a great extent been lifted. The sufferings undergone by millions of women through the centuries no longer had to be borne by their successors, at least in developed countries. It was a massive triumph for all womankind. There might be sorrow in the bearing of children, but there was now, for the first time, no need for nearly unbearable pain.

The haemorrhages

By 1900 the various forms of bleeding associated with pregnancy and birth had been categorized as:

1.   antepartum, divided into unavoidable and accidental; and,
2.   post-partum, after the delivery of the baby.

Unavoidable haemorrhage

PLACENTA PRAEVIA

As Edward Rigby (1747–1821) had pointed out in 1775 haemorrhage at some time before the birth of the baby was unavoidable when the placenta was attached to the lower part of the uterus. This is the part, later called the lower uterine segment, which stretches, rather than contracts as the upper segment does in labour. Such stretching, or giving way before the presenting part of the baby, is a necessary accompaniment of delivery. It may occur some few weeks before the onset of labour as the presenting part settles into the pelvis. It is certain to occur as the woman goes into labour. The placenta itself is inextensible. When its bed is stretched it must separate from its attachments and this tears across the maternal blood vessels at the site.

The time of onset of the bleeding in pregnancy is very variable, though by definition some time after 28 weeks. Its characteristic is that it is painless and repeated. It is repeated since the lower segment may stretch only slightly on several occasions during pregnancy allowing clotting to occur in the intervals, so temporarily preventing further bleeding. On the other hand bleeding may initially be extremely severe. The clinical presentation is therefore very variable too. The loss of blood may seem trivial at first, but it can suddenly become torrential and life-threatening. It is always a potentially terrifying event for all concerned.

In earlier centuries, and even in the earlier decades of the 20th century the problem was to know what to do about it, especially when the bleeding was severe. Justine Siegemundin (1650–1705), the celebrated German midwife, advocated, along with Mauriceau and others, that the membranes should be ruptured. This can be of value in some cases for it may allow the presenting part to be firmly pressed against the placenta and its bed and that may stem the bleeding. When the breech presented a leg was brought down and pulled on so that the baby's bottom pressed against the placenta. Of course, the older obstetricians performed internal version to convert a head presentation to breech for the same purpose. Another, virtually useless, method was to pack the vagina as tightly as possible. It probably only hid the bleeding from sight. But it might have had some value if the uterus contracted, for then there could be counter pressure on the placenta between the head and the pack.

These were still the only methods used until the early 20th century. Then caesarean section became more possible because of safer anaesthesia. But the operation still caused great anxiety. John Martin Munro Kerr (1868–1960) of Glasgow, and the doyen of British obstetrics, was opposed to caesarean section for placenta praevia in 1902. He probably then represented accepted practice. Up to 1910 in the United Kingdom the operation had only been performed seven times for this condition. By 1909 Munro Kerr had performed a section for placenta praevia and seven years later he had done only three. Even in 1933 he sounded warnings against the too free use of caesarean section. As far on as 1950 he still advocated internal version and plugging with the half breech in some cases. He also thought that if version could not be performed then the vagina should be tightly packed with a long cloth.

These approaches can be understood when it is known that in 1844 James Young Simpson found that the maternal mortality in placenta praevia was 30 per cent and the fetal mortality 60 per cent when using these methods. Even with some increasing use of caesarean section Comyns Berkeley in London in 1936 had a maternal mortality of seven per cent and a fetal mortality of 59 per cent. In 1939 Francis J. Browne of London still had maternal deaths in 5.9 per cent of his cases and fetal deaths in 54 per cent. He was using caesarean section when necessary.

It was Browne who tried more closely to define the indications for various forms of treatment in placenta praevia. On digital vaginal examination, always under general anaesthesia, he classified four grades of placenta praevia. They were:

1. when the placental edge only just encroached on the lower uterine segment;
2. when the edge of the placenta reached just to the orifice of the internal os of the cervix;
3. when the placenta partially covered the os but would be pulled out of the way as the lower segment was drawn upwards; and,
4. when the placenta covered the internal os completely and would never be pulled away from in front of the presenting part.

It became part of the routine never to examine vaginally any woman who had any bleeding in the latter half of pregnancy. In several cases it had been found that such examinations separated the placenta even more from its bed and could precipitate torrential bleeding. Any vaginal examination had therefore to be undertaken under anaesthesia in a fully equipped operating theatre ready to proceed to caesarean section forthwith, in case of severe haemorrhage.

Obviously enough a Grade 4 placenta praevia required caesarean section. There was no other way to effect delivery safely. Grade 3 too, more often than not, needed caesarean section despite the theoretical possibility that delivery could come about with the head passing the placenta by, compressing it in the meantime. In Grade 1 the woman could be left to go into labour as a result of the rupture of the membranes, which had to be done to be able to feel the placenta through the cervix. Grade 2 was probably safe to leave to vaginal delivery, but even in those cases everything had to be ready for a caesarean section at a moment's notice, for bleeding could be severe at any time.

The pattern of care was finally established by Professor C.H.G. Macafee and Joyce Morgan in Belfast in 1955. All patients with any vaginal bleeding in later pregnancy had to be admitted to hospital for observation, and kept there until delivery. The idea was to be ready to perform a caesarean section at any time if the bleeding became severe. But the main objective was to allow time for the fetus to grow towards maturity when its life would then be in lesser danger from prematurity. This waiting policy was abandoned by caesarean section if the bleeding became threatening to the mother. When the baby was thought to be mature enough the woman was examined vaginally in an operating theatre to try to determine how to proceed, by inducing labour or performing a section.

This policy reduced the maternal mortality to 0.3 per cent and the fetal mortality to 12 per cent. This was good enough vindication for the policy to be accepted universally. It had the drawback that many vaginal bleeds in pregnancy were subsequently found not to be due to placenta praevia. In the event they turned out to be quite innocuous. Yet the woman might have been confined to bed in hospital for many months, and that was only later found to have been unnecessary. But there was at that time no sure way to diagnose the presence of placenta praevia other than by vaginal clinical examination. This could be very dangerous except under the circumstances enumerated above.

Clinically it might be guessed that if the head was not engaged in the pelvis at term, then the placenta might be in front of the head, but this is a totally unreliable sign. The head may be high for a variety of other reasons. For a time it was thought that posterior placenta praevia could be diagnosed clinically by pressing the head backwards and counting the fetal heart rate. It was argued that this pressure reduced the placental blood flow which caused slowing of the fetal heart. But it turned out that it was the pressure on the head raising the intracranial pressure which was the cause of slowing. It occurred wherever the placenta was situated.

It was therefore essential to seek reliable methods of antenatal diagnosis so that those who did not have a placenta praevia were not subjected to the onerous hospital regime of staying in bed, waiting for term and for the baby to mature. The obvious way then to find the site of the placenta in the uterus was by some form of radiology.

In 1933 Munro Kerr and W.G. Mackay had injected a radio-opaque dye into the amniotic cavity. The intention was to show a filling defect in the shadow of the cavity where the placenta would be. But the method sometimes precipitated labour and there might be deleterious effects on the fetus. There had to be several exposures with the woman in different positions under the X-ray tube. Another method was to introduce the radio-opaque dye into the bladder (cystography). If the fetal head outline was always more than 1" away from the shadow of the dye then it was probable that the placenta intervened between them and was therefore in the anterior part of the lower uterine segment – a placenta praevia. But, of course, this could only diagnose an anterior praevia. All other types would be missed.

In 1934 W. Snow and C.B. Powell of America introduced soft tissue radiography without the use of dyes. Late in pregnancy the placenta might show small areas of calcification which show up on the radiograph. Of course these do not always define the lower edge of the placenta, so placenta praevia could not necessarily be excluded by this sign. However if the calcification was definitely in the upper segment of the uterus then placenta praevia was unlikely.

More than this though it was claimed that the placenta could actually be visualized on the plain X-ray. The outline of the uterus and the back of the baby may sometimes easily be seen. If they are close to one another then the placenta cannot intervene. There were also soft tissue shadows which were said to be showing the outline of the placenta, especially when it was seen 'on edge', for then one was looking through the whole substance of the organ. However, it was later realized that the liquor amnii itself could show a 'layered' appearance which could easily be mistaken for the placenta. At best soft tissue radiography was unreliable. Clinicians could not safely act on its findings.

A little later a better technique was found to be intra-arterial injection of radio-opaque dye into the femoral artery. The vascular tree of the uterus and the placenta were easily visible and a sure diagnosis of placenta praevia could be made. But it seemed an alarming way to establish the diagnosis. Sometimes there was arterial bleeding of some severity from the puncture of the artery. Finally all these methods gave way to firm diagnosis by the use of ultrasound, which is non-invasive, causing little disturbance of the patient, and being very accurate.

It was, of course, blood transfusion and the development of chemotherapy and antibiotics that made it possible to use caesarean section more freely for placenta praevia. Both subjects are dealt with later.

Accidental haemorrhage

ABRUPTIO PLACENTAE

Accidental haemorrhage was the term used by Edward Rigby for haemorrhages from the placental site when that was normally situated in the upper segment of the uterus. He believed that sometimes the placenta separated from its bed as a result of abdominal trauma. This can happen but is very rare. The name can be misleading, so Oliver Wendell Holmes suggested *ablatio placentae*. But it became better known as *abruptio placentae* after Joseph Bolivar De Lee (1869–1942) of Chicago so named it. It is excellently expressive in describing the tearing away of the placenta from the uterine wall. The woman feels a searing pain in the abdomen in the worst cases, and that, with extensive internal bleeding leads to shock, shown by pallor, coldness, sweating, raised pulse rate and low blood pressure, and then diminished urine output. Even to the casual observer it is a serious emergency. That is when there is massive internal bleeding, and this became known as *concealed* accidental haemorrhage. There could be lesser bleeds and then there might be some bleeding through the cervix and down the vagina. This was called *revealed* accidental haemorrhage. There were varying degrees of abdominal or back pain even with this lesser syndrome.

This distinction between concealed and revealed was over-elaborate. What mattered was the general state of the mother and the fate of the baby. Whether the bleeding was mainly internal or slightly external was of no great significance. It was the effect of the blood loss on the mother that mattered, and on her baby. But it took time for many obstetricians to realize these facts. The cause of the disorder was not known then, and is not known now, although theories abound. The main cause was thought to be toxaemia of pregnancy, as it was called. It had been noted that after the event many of these abruption patients had albumin in the urine, which is one characteristic of toxaemia. Although such patients have low blood pressure due to the haemorrhage it was postulated that it had been high, as if it were pushing the placenta off its bed by its force. However, wartime experience showed that severely injured soldiers, with massive haemorrhage, often also developed albuminuria. So this sign could be an effect of bleeding rather than a part of its cause. Another fact ignored by this toxaemia theory was that almost never did patients with severe accidental haemorrhage show signs of toxaemia – raised blood pressure, albuminuria and oedema – prior to the catastrophe.

The nature of this disaster began to be understood a little better in 1911 when Alexandre Couvelaire (1873–1948) of Paris performed a caesarean section, under chloroform, on a woman with accidental haemorrhage, whose condition was rapidly deteriorating. He was amazed by what he saw. The uterus was purple due to blood in its wall, and there was some blood in the peritoneal cavity. The placenta was free in a uterus full of blood and clot. He thought the uterus would never recover from what looked like gangrene, so he removed it together with the tubes and ovaries, and in effect performed a Porro caesarean section. In all such cases he recommended that this should be done and his advice was widely followed. He described the condition as uterine apoplexy. The treatment was drastic but was probably right for the time and may have saved many maternal lives at the expense of total loss of further reproductive function.

Towards the middle of the century it was usual to pursue a waiting policy in these cases. As always, of course, bleeding from the uterus is controlled by delivery of the baby and the placenta, thus allowing muscular contraction to close the maternal blood vessels at the placental site, this to be followed by clotting in the mouths of the vessels for more permanent arrest of bleeding. The obvious choice was to rupture the membranes, hoping the woman would go into labour as quickly as possible. In milder cases this did often happen, and because so little of the placenta had separated the baby frequently survived too. It became accepted that up to one-third of the placenta might separate without necessarily destroying the fetus through anoxia.

The older obstetricians were impressed by the fact that rupturing the membranes in severe accidental haemorrhage was frequently not followed by labour for some time. They said that the uterus was paralysed and unable to contract. This was a misinterpretation since the uterus in these cases is always rock hard to the touch, showing it to be in fact in a state of tonic contraction. Rupturing the membranes restores polarity, and that can be aided by a pitocin drip, so bringing on labour. Again the older obstetricians were misled into thinking the uterus would not contract properly by the fact that cases of accidental haemorrhage often have post-partum haemorrhage too. For them the only cause of post-partum haemorrhage was a relaxed inefficient uterus which would not contract properly. It was only later that it was realized that such post-partum haemorrhage is due to failure of clotting – *afibrinogenaemia* as it was then called. The massive haemorrhage everywhere caused gross depletion of the essential ingredient of fibrinogen in clotting. The bleeding continued however well the uterus contracted in the third stage.

A further complication that was not fully understood at first was total renal failure. It was due to prolonged hypotension, which was erroneously allowed to persist because of inadequate blood transfusion. It was not a failure of the kidney substance but of its circulation. There seemed to be a general reluctance to transfuse adequate amounts of blood in obstetrics. It was thought that massive transfusion would bring back the hypertension which had been postulated but not proven. The lessons of military trauma fortunately changed this reluctance.

About the mid-century the proper policy to pursue became clearer. First pain had to be relieved by adequate injections of morphine. A minimum of two pints of blood was transfused, and then further amounts were given until pulse, blood pressure and skin colour returned, watching all the time for signs of over-transfusion as shown by raised venous pressure in the neck. If the baby was alive, which was unusual, then caesarean section had to be considered. However, even when that was done the baby often died soon after birth since it had been rendered irredeemably anoxic before birth. So, commonly the membranes were ruptured. The cervix was always partially dilated and the membranes bulging, showing that the uterus was contracting and raising the pressure within it. Labour supervened quickly but could be aided by an oxytocin drip if there was delay. Provided this policy was pursued correctly the results for the mother improved immensely. She was spared long painful delay waiting for natural labour to begin. Adequate blood transfusion prevented renal shut-down. A watch was kept for clotting defects. There came to be several types of these depending on which factors in the clotting mechanism had been depleted. Haematologists were then able to supply the appropriate remedy for intravenous infusion. At first it was thought that the depletion was always of fibrinogen. It was only when infusions of this, as quadruple strength plasma, sometimes failed that further research showed there were about 14 factors involved in clotting, as in a form of cascade, one part of the mechanism being followed by another until firm clot formed.

Post-partum haemorrhage

Some bleeding after the birth of the baby is to be expected as the placenta separates from its bed and is delivered in the third stage of labour. Maternal blood vessels are inevitably torn. During this period of the 20th century the definition of post-partum haemorrhage (PPH) was a loss of one pint or more of blood. Of course it was always wisest to prevent so much blood being lost. It was done by rubbing up a contraction by massaging the uterus through the abdominal wall. Then when it was sure that the placenta had been expelled from the uterine cavity, as shown by the uterus changing its shape, rising up in the abdomen and becoming mobile, the placenta was pushed out of the vagina by pressing downwards on the uterus, using it as a sort of plunger. This was essentially the method advocated by John Harvie in the 18th century.

If the placenta remained inside the uterus and bleeding continued then Carl Credé's (1819–1892) method of squeezing the uterus between the two hands on the abdomen was often advocated. It could be both shocking and ineffective. Failing that there had to be recourse to manual removal. Although this had been used for centuries it was avoided as much as possible at this period for it could increase shock and introduce infection. The shock was, however, somewhat diminished by always performing the operation under general anaesthesia and by blood transfusion which was often necessary. Later chemotherapy and antibiotics diminished anxiety about infection. Liquid extract of ergot was given by mouth after delivery of the placenta, by whatever means, normal or assisted, in order to make the uterus contract. Its action was delayed because of the oral administration and the extract varied in the strength of its active principles. Then in 1935 J. Chassar Moir (1900–1977), then in London, and Harold Ward Dudley (1887–1935) isolated ergometrine from ergot. This was much more effective than ergotoxine which Henry Hallett Dale (1875–1966) had isolated in 1906, and ergotamine extracted by Karl Spiro (1867–1932) and Arthur Stoll (1887–1971) in 1918.

Ergometrine came to be widely used by injection after the placenta had been delivered. It caused almost immediate contraction of the uterus. It was not at first given before delivery of the placenta for it was thought that it might cause the formation of a constriction ring which would imprison the placenta making it difficult to deliver, even by manual removal. But just before 1950 this was shown to be untrue. Chassar Moir suggested the use of a small dose of ergometrine intravenously (0.125 mgm.) as the baby's head was being born (crowning). The idea was that the body of the baby within the uterus would prevent the development of a constriction ring. The treatment was highly effective and reduced the PPH rate from about 10 per cent to about 3 per cent or lower. Later the dose of ergometrine was increased to 0.5 mgm.

The results were better still when oxytocin (Syntocinon), which had now been obtained in pure form synthetically, was given at the same time as the ergometrine. Oxytocin causes immediate contraction while ergometrine prolongs the duration of the contracted state. The combined drug was called Syntometrine. This became used worldwide. Almost invariably the placenta was separated from the uterine wall immediately after the birth of the baby and it came to lie in the lower uterine segment or upper part of the vagina. It then became routine to draw the placenta out of the birth canal by pulling gently on the umbilical cord (a time-honoured method), while at the same time lifting the uterus upwards into the abdomen with a hand just above the symphysis pubis. The placenta was held by its cord while the uterus was lifted upwards off it. This is still standard treatment. It has reduced the incidence of PPH to very low proportions. It marked yet another milestone in making childbirth much safer than it had ever been before.

Blood transfusion

The safe transfusion of whole blood transformed the prognosis of all types of haemorrhage in midwifery practice. Before the 20th century it is probable that millions of women must have died from obstetric haemorrhages. Attempts had been made from as early as the 17th century to transfuse blood. A transfusion between two people was successfully carried out in London in 1667 by Richard Lower (1631–1691) and Edmund King (1629–1707). They were obviously lucky for there are many technical and biological problems to be solved, of which they could not have known. The first is how to prevent clotting when blood is collected. Braxton Hicks of Guy's Hospital tried sodium phosphate. James Blundell (1790–1877) of the same hospital treated a patient with postpartum haemorrhage by pouring blood into a funnel connected by tubing to a needle entering a vein.

A biological problem is that not all bloods are compatible with one another. Mismatched transfusions, disrupting red blood cells, may cause anxiety, breathlessness, pain in the chest, a bursting feeling in the head, surgical shock and later renal failure perhaps leading to death. Some understanding of these disasters came when Karl Landsteiner (1868–1943) in 1900 showed the presence of iso-agglutinins in many bloods. If incompatible blood is transfused these iso-agglutinins in serum haemolyse the foreign blood, and it is the haemoglobin so released from the red cells which causes the problems enumerated above. Further work showed the four major blood groups, now well-known as O, A, B and AB. The cells carry agglutinogens which can excite immune responses when injected into others. Group O blood serum contains anti-A and anti-B and no agglutinogens; A anti-B and A agglutinogens; B anti-A and B agglutinogens; AB has no iso-agglutinins but both A and B agglutinogens. Group O people are universal donors, able to have their blood transfused into all others. Group AB are universal recipients, able to receive blood of any group from others. Further detail is unnecessary here. The important thing was to match the corpuscles of the donor with the serum of the recipient.

In practice this was earlier done by the clinician himself mixing some serum from the recipient with a drop of blood from the donor on a microscope slide. Agglutination of the blood cells was easily seen by the naked eye in the incompatible bloods. When there was compatibility there was no such clumping. But later the iso-agglutinins were specially prepared and cross-matching of blood became a laboratory procedure, but this was not universally so until near the middle of the century. Now cross-matching is always performed in the haematological laboratories and has been automated.

An advance in safety was made when Richard Lewisohn (1875–1962), in the USA, used sodium citrate to prevent clotting in blood taken from a donor. Oswald Hope Robertson (1886–1966) used such treated stored blood in battle casualties in 1917–1918. By 1935 Hugh Leslie Marriott (1900–1983) and Alan Kekwick (1909–1974) of the Middlesex Hospital, London, introduced the slow drip method of transfusion, which is now universal. It greatly increased safety. Previously, massive rapid transfusions could overwhelm the circulation and cause cardiac failure.

In 1935 the first blood bank in the world was established in Chicago by Bernard Fantus (1874–1940). This was made possible by sodium citrate and refrigeration. Such stored fluid blood could be used for two to three weeks after it had been taken from donors. Such was the need for blood transfusion in the war of 1939–45 that the National Blood Transfusion Service was set up in the United Kingdom. It still exists and is able to supply large quantities of blood, and now blood products, to all hospitals for a variety of purposes. Naturally the important knowledge of the value of transfusion gained in the treatment of wartime trauma was quickly imported into obstetric practice with immensely beneficial effects, in all forms of haemorrhage.

Despite all known precautions being taken to match donor and recipient bloods carefully, there were still some unexplained transfusion reactions. In 1940 some of these were shown to be due to the Rhesus factor by Karl Landsteiner and Alexander Solomon Wiener (b.1907), of the USA. Apart from blood transfusion this discovery came to have great importance for midwifery in ways previously unsuspected. It was recognized as the cause of *erythroblastosis fetalis* by Philip Levine (b.1900) in 1941.

About 85 per cent of women are Rhesus positive, which means that their blood is agglutinated by serum obtained from Rhesus monkeys. The other 15 per cent are Rhesus negative. Their cells are not agglutinated by Rhesus serum. In certain circumstances, now well-defined, but to be taken up later, a Rhesus negative woman bearing a Rhesus positive fetus may manufacture antibodies to the fetal blood. The antibodies may then cross the placenta and by haemolysis destroy large quantities of the baby's blood. Depending on the degree of anaemia so caused the baby may be born anaemic and after birth develop jaundice which can damage the brain; or it may die in utero of severe cardiac failure which expresses itself as massive oedema and death in the condition called *hydrops fetalis*.

The development of safe transfusion meant that yet another scourge of childbearing was largely defeated. In well-equipped surroundings in the western world no woman was now likely to die inevitably as a result of blood loss. That had been the case for vast numbers until the second quarter of the 20th century.

Puerperal fever

The major killers of childbearing women through the centuries have been haemorrhage and infection. After the birth of the placenta there is a large open wound on the inner surface of the uterus. Micro-organisms can easily gain access to it through the vagina and cervix. If birth has been traumatic with lacerations lower down the genital tract, infections there readily climb up to the placental site. Spread of infection from there may be to the Fallopian tubes or through the uterine wall to the peritoneum, or be more widely disseminated through the rich plexus of veins and lymphatics of the placental bed.

It is more often than not the attendants at birth who carry infection to the woman. This was decisively shown by White, Gordon, Semmelweis and Wendell Holmes. Pasteur showed that the cause of puerperal fever was bacteria, often streptococci. Lister demonstrated the importance of antisepsis as well as asepsis. These were the major tools of prevention of puerperal sepsis. Cure, when infection was established, was much more difficult to achieve before the coming of chemotherapy and antibiotic therapy. Until they came the treatment had to be bed rest, change of diet, and nursing care in the hope that the body's defences would ultimately triumph over the invaders. That could take a long time, and recovery was often accompanied by widespread abscesses, deep thrombosis of the leg veins and chronic inflammation in the pelvis leading to debilitating gynaecological disorders.

Original attempts to cure infectious diseases were made by Louis Pasteur when he inoculated a boy infected with rabies. This was in 1885. In 1891 Emil von Behring (1854–1917) successfully treated diphtheria with an antitoxin. The idea arose that treatment should be directed to stimulating antibody production by a variety of vaccines. Antibodies are chemical and so they were called 'humoral'. In addition there were realized to be 'cellular' mechanisms called into being to combat infection. These are mainly the white cells which ingest foreign materials in the process of phagocytosis described by Elie Metchnikoff (1845–1916) of Russia in 1895. In 1904 Sir Almroth Edward Wright (1861–1947) and Stewart Ranken Douglas (1871–1936) of London showed that phagocytosis was assisted by 'opsonins' which are humoral substances, so there was apparent combination of humoral and cellular immunity.

The first hint of the possibility of direct attack on infecting organisms came with the discovery of salvarsan in 1909, by Paul Ehrlich (1854–1915) and his assistant Sahachiro Hata (1873–1938), for the treatment of syphilis. Four years earlier Fritz Richard Schaudinn (1871–1906) and Paul Erich Hoffmann (1868–1959), zoologists of Berlin, had discovered and stained the causative organism of syphilis, which they called the *Treponema pallida*. In 1906 August von Wassermann (1866–1925) and Albert Neisser (1855–1916) had published their work on a blood test which showed whether a person had been infected with syphilis. This test was modified by Reuben Leon Kahn (b.1887) of Chicago in 1922. With all this work, especially that of Ehrlich, chemotherapy became a perceived reality. His research was phenomenal and painstaking. Salvarsan was not discovered until 606 experiments had been conducted to find a drug for the treatment of syphilis.

It was Gerhard Domagk (1895–1964) who, in 1935, discovered the value of a dye called *Prontosil rubrum* in the treatment of acute bacterial infections. It was found to contain sulphanilamide. Rapidly many other sulphonamides were produced and they formed a massive armamentarium against a variety of infections, often caused by streptococci and staphylococci. These were the commonest causes of puerperal infections. Almost overnight the prognosis for these formerly dire infections was transformed. Whereas women with puerperal fever were frequently ill for a long time and not too uncommonly died they were now cured in a day or two by one or other of the sulphonamide drugs.

An immense amount of bacteriological work was done on the varieties of streptococci, including the anaerobic kind, and the staphylococci during the 1930s and 1940s. Then in 1929 penicillin was discovered by Alexander Fleming (1881–1955). Its therapeutic qualities were, however, not appreciated until 1940 when Ernest Boris Chain (1906–1979) and Howard Florey (1898–1968) used it in Oxford. At that time it had to be injected, often three-hourly. It was so remarkable in combating acute infection, such as occurred in war wounds, that as soon as enough of it could be manufactured it came into universal use. It too transformed the scene in cases of puerperal sepsis, as well as many other infectious diseases caused by bacteria.

Then the floodgates of antibiotic therapy opened and there came streptomycin (1944), chloramphenicol (1947), aureomycin (1948), cephalosporin (1948), neomycin (1949), terramycin (1950) and a host of others. In all but a few cases of bacterial obstetric infections cure became the rule. Another scourge of childbearing women had been almost completely vanquished. Bacteria causing disease could be categorised and identified in the laboratory and the appropriate antibiotics determined so that therapy became more or less specific for each person. More often than not it was efficacious too. It was a great triumph of scientific and clinical medicine, and achieved in the course of about 70 years from the beginnings of bacteriology.

Pregnancy

The toxaemias of pregnancy

In the first half of the 20th century there were some disorders arising in pregnancy which were not understood but were assumed to be due to toxins. This was a prevalent belief used to explain a variety of medical and surgical conditions. It has been shown to be quite unsubstantiated as regards midwifery.

Hyperemesis gravidarum

Some unfortunate women in early pregnancy do not simply suffer from 'morning sickness' which is common, they have severe repeated excessive vomiting. Once established it can lead on to physical signs in the central nervous system. These are nystagmus (a form of twitching of the eyeballs), psychological changes, as well as liver and renal failure, sometimes causing death. The psychosis was described by the Russian Sergei Sergeyevich Korsakoff (1854–1900) and named after him. There is loss of memory for recent events, disorientation and confabulation. This last means that the patient invents stories about herself which are patently untrue to others but which she believes to be true. It can occur in alcoholism too.

Only about the middle of the century did it become apparent that the initial nausea was in some way related to the rising amounts of hormones in the blood, coming from the placenta. Why this should advance to excessive vomiting was less clear, but tended to be attributed to psychological causes, perhaps an unconscious rejection of pregnancy. But in the fourth and fifth decades it did become obvious that the ill effects of the vomiting were caused by water and salt depletion, and vitamin deficiency.

Owen Harding Wangensteen (1898–1981) published a paper in 1932 about fluid and electrolyte balances in surgery, and particularly in intestinal obstruction. Slowly there came appreciation of the importance of water and salt balance in many aspects of surgery. Just as slowly the appreciation spread into obstetric practice. Virtually all the clinical phenomena of hyperemesis gravidarum were explicable in terms of water and salt depletion caused by the vomiting and the consequent loss of fluid and electrolytes from the stomach and intestinal secretions. By the mid-century the treatment was replacement of fluid and electrolyte losses by intravenous infusions, supplemented with vitamin therapy, mainly of the B group. The technique was to measure the total output of fluid from bowel, bladder and skin, the latter being estimated. Enough fluid was given to replace these losses and to restore the daily urine volume to normal. Blood electrolytes were monitored in the chemical pathology laboratories and the composition of the infusion fluid was altered as necessary to restore the chemical composition of the blood to normal.

This symptomatic therapy was entirely successful, despite the cause being unknown. Patients recovered where formerly they had died, as Charlotte Brontë had done. After its introduction there was rarely necessity for termination of pregnancy which had earlier been the only known treatment. Strangely the disorder became much less common. This may be because of the introduction of some medicines which reduce nausea and perhaps because of different culturally perceived approaches to the psychology of childbearing.

Eclampsia

Earlier the only known characteristic of this malady was fits, occurring in the second half of pregnancy or during the first week or so of the puerperium. The fits came suddenly and were said to flash out, which is the meaning of the word eclampsia. Some premonitory symptoms and signs of fits were spots before the eyes, headache, and jaundice due to liver failure, and anuria due to renal failure. In 1843 Lever of Guy's Hospital, London, had shown that after the fits many women had albumin in the urine. This seemed to suggest that the disorder was similar to Bright's disease of the kidneys.

Several attempts were made to measure blood pressure during the 19th century, but no instruments were simple enough to use clinically until the introduction of the sphygmomanometer in 1896 by Scipione Riva-Rocci (1863–1937) of Turin, in a form similar to that still known and used today. It took some time for it to be universally used in midwifery, but when it was realized that a feature of toxaemia of pregnancy was a raised blood pressure the sphygmomanometer came into routine use in pregnancy, labour and the puerperium.

In 1905 Nikolai Sergeivich Korotkoff (1874–1920) of Russia described the sounds to be heard through a stethoscope placed over the brachial artery after the sphygmomanometer cuff had been inflated above the systolic pressure and then slowly released. The first sound is a tapping noise in time with the pulse, and this is taken to be the systolic pressure. The sounds then become louder and louder and then become muffled, and this point is taken as the diastolic reading on the falling mercury column. Finally the sounds disappear entirely. There is still some argument about which sound is best taken as the diastolic pressure, the muffling or the disappearance.

The dramatic event is eclampsia, or fits, whenever they occur. Vassili Vassilievich Stroganoff (1857–1938) of Russia first successfully treated them and reduced their dire prognosis. He wrote about his treatment in 1897 but the methods were not described in English until 1930. He wrote:

> 'The object which the prophylactic method has is to interrupt the fits by acting on the patient with all the means and measures we have at our disposal. In removing the fits we at the same time remove the vascular spasm, and thus

119

contribute in bringing the pregnant or parturient woman to a normal condition or to a state of pre-eclamptic toxaemia. In removing the fits we decrease the output of new toxins, which, in addition to the previous ones, serve to increase their destructive power.'

It is interesting to note his reference to vascular spasm because hypertension is essentially due to that, for it raises the peripheral resistance. He was still imprisoned though by the belief in toxins as the cause of the spasm and the fits.

His method consisted of removing all forms of stimulation of the patient from the room. All noise was to be avoided. Light was excluded. Physical examinations, especially vaginal, were to be reduced to an absolute minimum. If they had to be done chloroform narcosis was administered. The same was needed for enemas and catheterization of the bladder. An attendant was to be in the room at all times, ready to administer chloroform if a further fit occurred. Oxygen had to be at the ready since anoxia during fits was common.

There was no doubt that almost any variety of stimulation would bring on a fit in a woman who had already had one. In addition to this regime, morphia injections were given under chloroform narcosis, followed by chloral hydrate by mouth. All this was done in a rigidly defined timed schedule. If there were signs indicating the possibility of a cerebral haemorrhage a caesarean section was to be done immediately. It was known that if fits could be prevented for about 12 hours then they were unlikely to recur.

Stroganoff also used venesection sometimes, removing 13oz of blood. It was probably of some value though he advocated using it very cautiously. He was doubtful too about the use of magnesium sulphate enemas which had some vogue in the USA. The intention there was to diminish the excitability of the brain, the proximate cause of the fits. Of course labour often supervened after the first fits. This was managed conservatively using chloroform narcosis as necessary to diminish the stimulation of the pains. Delivery of the baby was by forceps under general anaesthesia. The full regime was continued for about 12 hours after the birth.

Stroganoff's results were a great improvement on what had gone before. Up to 1918 his maternal mortality was about five per cent. During the same period treatment by other methods in other hands were in the region of 20–25 per cent. Watts Eden in 1922 analysed the results from 15 London teaching hospitals in the period from 1911 to 1921. In 547 cases there had been a mortality of 22.1 per cent. When coma was a complication the mortality rose to 34 per cent, and if the coma were deep it was 63 per cent. Later Stroganoff's mortality rose to ten per cent in his 141 cases. Then he analysed 2,495 cases of eclampsia in Europe from 1924 to 1929 when there were 250 deaths, a mortality of ten per cent, where his methods had been used.

Stroganoff seems not at first to have recognized the importance of raised blood pressure in what became known as pre-eclamptic toxaemia, nor even in his cases of eclampsia itself. But Watts Eden and his collaborators about 1924 knew that the prognosis in eclampsia worsened if the blood pressure rose to more than 200 mmHg, and also if the temperature rose to 103° Fahrenheit. This shows that the sphygmomanometer was coming into increasing use in the 1920s and 1930s, but not much before that. But in the English edition of his book of 1930 Stroganoff did know about blood pressure. He wrote:

'The forerunners of fits are: increase of headache [which is recognizable in unconscious patients by the expression of the face, restlessness in bed], convulsive contractions of separate muscles, dimming of vision, and especially increase of blood pressure.'

The Stroganoff method of treating patients with fits is still practised in its essentials though the drugs used vary from place to place and from time to time. By the mid-century however the emphasis had changed from controlling fits to preventing them ever occurring by the vigilance of ante-natal care. The idea of the disorder being due to toxins was gradually abandoned and this hypertensive toxaemia of pregnancy was increasingly called pre-eclampsia. It denotes an illness which may lead to eclampsia if untreated. This is descriptive rather than implying knowledge of the underlying aetiology.

This work was another milestone in making childbirth much safer than it had been.

Antenatal care

It is presently impossible to comprehend how pregnancy and its problems were almost completely ignored by professionals. Yet it was not until the 20th century that any serious notice of it was taken. In some ways the former neglect can be understood. By contrast with pregnancy, labour is dramatic and sometimes attended by sudden and serious problems which demand immediate intervention. Some complications of pregnancy are similarly demanding, but pregnancy is a quieter slower process than labour.

It was in 1901 that John William Ballantyne (1861–1923) of Edinburgh published in the *British Medical Journal* an article called, 'A Plea for a Pro-maternity Hospital'. He referred to the ignorance surrounding eclampsia, hyperemesis gravidarum, jaundice, hydramnios (excessive amounts of fluid round the fetus), hydatidiform mole (a tumour of the placenta), diseases of the fetus, the causes of fetal death, maternal physiology, the urine, the blood, the origin of the liquor amnii, placental function and the physiology of the fetus. This was a masterly comprehensive analysis of the problems yet to be solved. It began to open the eyes of professionals to vistas which they had never before seen or contemplated. For the first time the fetus was accorded some clinical status, which it had never had previously. The mother had always taken precedence whenever the interests of mother and baby clashed.

Ballantyne wrote:

'Of course the foetal heart was listened to and a few conclusions drawn therefrom and there was a certain degree of accuracy in the palpation of the foetal parts; but antenatal diagnosis was far from exact and it was indeed little attempted ...

The question may fairly be asked if we of the twentieth century are going to be contented with the knowledge or ignorance of the nineteenth in these matters of the physiology and pathology of pregnancy.'

Ballantyne's proposal for a Pro-maternity Hospital was 'for the reception of women who are pregnant but who are not yet in labour'. He expected that some of these would have had problems in previous childbearing episodes. Also he hoped to help some in 'whose present condition some anomaly of the pregnant state has been diagnosed'.

'.... practically no provision is made in existing hospitals for pregnant women. In general hospitals cases of morbid pregnancy (for example hyperemesis gravidarum) are sometimes received and treated, but mostly under protest lest there occur a birth in the wards.'

Such protests still occur.

As a result of his energy one bed was endowed by another Edinburgh obstetrician, Freeland Barbour. It was called the Alexander Hamilton bed after a previous professor of obstetrics. Quite quickly the number of beds increased to four, and later still to 25. For etymological reasons pro-maternity was changed to pre-maternity.

Ballantyne did not attempt to provide an out-patient service for pregnant women. This was done in Boston, Mass., in 1901, where some antenatal visits were made to women in their own homes. The visits were made by members of the Instructive Nursing Association. By 1906 all women booked to have their babies in the Boston Lying-in Hospital were visited at least once during pregnancy. By 1912 all received three visits from nurses. In 1909 Mrs William Lowell Putnam of the Infant Social Service Department of the Women's Municipal League of Boston instituted intensive care of pregnant women. They were visited at home every ten days and given advice about pregnancy and its hygiene. In 1911 the Lying-in Hospital set up an antenatal department within its walls.

In 1913 Ballantyne also established a domiciliary out-patient department in Edinburgh and a hospital out-patient clinic in 1915. Similar arrangements were made in Adelaide, South Australia, by Thomas George Wilson and in Sydney by J.C. Windeyer in 1910. The value of the new idea was obviously appreciated widely. In 1918 in England and Wales the Maternity and Child Welfare Act gave powers to Local Authorities to set up antenatal clinics and to provide dental care in pregnancy, as well as to offer milk and food to indigent women at reduced prices. Childbearing increased in political importance because of the carnage of the 1914–1918 war in which over one million young men of the United Kingdom died. It was felt that those who had died should be replaced by more births.

Local Authority clinics numbered 120 in 1918. By 1944 there were 1,931. In 1950 it was estimated that there were 2,000 clinics supervising the care of 73 per cent of all expectant mothers. An investigation of 1946, just after the war of 1939–45, by the Royal College of Obstetricians and Gynaecologists together with the Population Investigation Committee found that only 0.9 per cent of mothers had not received any antenatal care at all. In 50 years the scene had changed from one of virtually no antenatal care to almost universal care in the UK.

Ballantyne had laid down the appropriate methods of antenatal care. A personal and family history was to be taken, and each woman was to be physically examined regularly. By the 1920s the blood pressure was regularly measured and the urine tested for albumin. In 1923 he wrote that the aims of antenatal care were:

1.   to remove dread;
2.   to reduce discomfort;
3.   to treat syphilis and pre-eclamptic toxaemia early;
4.   to increase the numbers of normal pregnancies and labours;
5.   to reduce the stillbirth rate; and,
6.   to reduce maternal mortality.

His emphasis on the psychology of pregnant women, at that early date, is noteworthy.

In 1932 Francis J. Browne of London criticized antenatal care for not achieving its original high aims. He pointed out that since 1911 there had been no fall in maternal deaths, nor in eclampsia, nor in stillbirths. The only change he could discern was in the reduction of cases of obstructed labour. It may be that this last was due to an increase in induction of premature labour. The criticism was not enough, however, to cause antenatal care to be discarded. It was not then recognized that many social factors were major contributors to maternal health. Later evidence does seem to show that maternal and fetal deaths and illnesses have fallen, partly as a result of antenatal care, though along with many other factors. There has been early diagnosis of intercurrent diseases, and some forewarning of potential problems of labour. The general consensus among professionals, and more importantly childbearing women themselves, seemed to be that antenatal care was valuable to them, even if statistical measurement did not always give them 'scientific' support.

By the 1940s the full routine of antenatal care had become established. At the first visit to the clinic a medical, surgical and obstetric history was taken and a complete clinical physical examination made. This included a vaginal examination. The intention here was to exclude abnormalities of the soft parts, such as ovarian cysts and fibroids, but also to estimate the size of the bony pelvis. This was described in great detail but there is no doubt that many clinicians misjudged their abilities to do this with accuracy. This was nicely demonstrated with the vogue for routine X-ray pelvimetry, when clinical assessments did not always accord with the radiological ones. Radiology does give accurate measurements, but not necessarily a reliable prognosis for labour and the possibility of obstruction. There are more factors in labour than simple sizes of fetal head and maternal pelvis.

The routine measurement of blood pressure and the clinical testing for oedema and for the presence of albumin in the urine were valuable for early recognition of pre-eclampsia and its treatment. Routine weighing added to the possibilities of detection of water retention, which might also be a sign of developing pre-eclampsia.

Unfortunately these examinations do not always detect the onset of pre-eclampsia, nor even of eclampsia. Yet they are better tools than anything else yet devised, so have to be used *faute de mieux*. The numbers of cases of eclampsia had fallen by the mid-century. Some of that fall must be attributed to antenatal care and the searches for raised blood pressure, albuminuria and oedema leading to early admission to hospital so that pre-eclampsia could be prevented from progressing to eclampsia.

Also important was the ability to test for syphilis with the Wassermann Reaction. Until the advent of penicillin this was a real scourge, causing, in the infected woman, repeated stillbirths, and if she did bear a live child it bore the stigmata of syphilis. These were saddle nose, notched teeth and general sickliness and failure to thrive.

Determination of the haemoglobin was valuable in the diagnosis and treatment of anaemia. This investigation led to the recognition that not only was iron deficiency microcytic anaemia common, but so also was a form of macrocytic anaemia specific to pregnancy and caused by folic acid deficiency. Lucy Wills (1888–1964) in 1931 showed that such macrocytic anaemia could be cured by yeast extracts. In 1946 folic acid was isolated from them as the active principle. Vitamin B12 was discovered to be the 'extrinsic factor' so being a part cause of pernicious anaemia when it was deficient. The blood group of each woman was determined. The usual blood groups were known so that if transfusion were necessary in emergency no time was wasted in cross matching. When the importance of the Rhesus factor in erythroblastosis fetalis was better understood its determination was helpful in saving babies from illness and death.

Another destructive disease of these times was pulmonary tuberculosis. Not only was it likely to deteriorate in pregnancy, but, if undetected, the mother might infect her baby after birth. Tuberculosis in babies can be rapidly fatal. Since the disease was so common and there was no specific treatment until streptomycin was discovered in 1944 by Albert Schatz et al, the disease was sought by routine chest X-rays, and bacteriology if necessary. Diagnosis allowed for sanatorium and other treatments and separation of the baby from its mother at birth. The baby could also be given BCG – Bacille-Calmette-Guèrin – in a form of immunization against the Mycobacterium tuberculosis. This had been introduced in 1927 by Léon Charles Albert Calmette (1863–1933) and others, including Camille Guèrin (1872–1961) of Paris.

Diabetes mellitus was also picked up early in pregnancy by routine testing of the urine for glucose. The disease may become more severe in pregnancy, but it also has serious effects in causing fetal abnormality and death, hydramnios, and large babies which can be a cause of difficult labour. Early effective treatment lowers the incidence of several of these disasters. Renal diseases, too, could be detected early in pregnancy if clinicians were alerted to the possibility by the presence of protein in the urine. It was important to treat renal disorder for the sake of the mother, but also because it could be a precursor of pre-eclampsia, which can be dangerous for the baby too.

In 1941 Norman McAlister Gregg (1892–1966) of Sydney, an ophthalmologist, discovered several children who suffered from cataract. Their mothers had all been affected by Rubella (German measles) in early pregnancy. This was an observation of far-reaching importance. Prior to this it had been assumed that all fetal and neonatal abnormalities were of genetic origin and therefore, for the times, undiagnosable, untreatable and not preventable. Now it was understood that the embryo and fetus were vulnerable to external, even slight, causes in the mother. By preventing exposure to rubella in early pregnancy or by acquired immunity in the mother's early childhood, or by vaccination, a variety of defects in neonates could perhaps be prevented. The defects included blindness, deafness, cardiac anomalies and mental retardation, all therefore serious yet caused by a normally mild maternal infection.

Ballantyne would have been delighted by the outcome of his ideas as they had developed. His appointment in Edinburgh was as a Lecturer in Antenatal Pathology and Teratology. One of his main aims had always been to prevent abnormalities in the fetus and newborn by caring for the mother. His vision was vindicated in 50 years. It required more advanced technology than he had had at his disposal. When that came his aspirations began to be fulfilled.

Antenatal care is therefore of value and became so in the first half of the 20th century. Its purely obstetric value was probably less than at first had been hoped. There was the chance to correct breech presentations and transverse lies by external version, but none of the other malpresentations and malpositions were amenable to treatment in pregnancy, though being forewarned of them might be valuable in the labour ward. It was helpful too to be forewarned of multiple pregnancy, fetal abnormality as shown on X-ray, and of the possibility of contracted pelvis and obstructed labour. But the real importance of antenatal care came with the recognition of intercurrent disorders, which might have their worst effects offset by early treatment for the benefit of both mother and baby. Antenatal care also provided opportunities for preparation of mothers for their own problems in labour and the puerperium by the methods of 'natural childbirth' teachings. Moreover they could be educated in matters of hygiene and diet which could be of value long after the birth.

Midwifery education and services
Midwives

The progress of earlier training and education of midwives and the qualification of LOS have been described in Chapter 9. As a result of many disparate initiatives the Midwives Act was passed through Parliament in 1902. It established the Central Midwives Board which was empowered to lay down training requirements for midwives, how long training should last, the supervision of examinations, and the holding of a Roll showing those who had fulfilled the requirements of the Board. The system was similar to that which had been put in place for doctors with the founding of the General Medical Council.

In 1905 the Roll of Midwives contained 22,308 names. The Licence of the Obstetrical Society of London (LOS) was held by 7,465 (33.5 per cent) of them, and a further 2,322 (ten per cent) held a certificate of training issued by a hospital. Another group of 12,521 (56 per cent) were adjudged to be *bona fide* midwives. They were deemed experienced enough to be admitted to the Roll even though they had not been formally trained. This was a good start.

An Act of 1910 made it an offence for anyone other than a registered midwife or doctor to attend a childbearing woman, except in an emergency. This was an excellent piece of legislation, providing some protection for women against unqualified amateurs. The same Act put the responsibility for midwifery care on to County Councils and County Borough Councils. Government at national and local levels was then fully concerned with proper midwife care for women. The Councils set up a Local Supervising Authority with a Midwifery Supervisor in charge. The Authorities employed some midwives but they also had regulatory control over midwives practising in their areas, whether in domiciliary or hospital practice, and whether practising privately or not.

In 1911 the Central Midwives Board decreed that all those on their Roll should regularly and frequently attend a revision course of lectures approved by them. This was a farsighted requirement and an early example of compulsory postgraduate continuing education. As regards the ordinary course to become a qualified midwife it was required that a generally trained nurse should undergo four months training, while others had to have six months. Usually the students had to pay for their courses themselves, since most midwifery was still in private hands.

In 1926 an Act for the registration and inspection of maternity homes by Local Authorities was passed. Midwives practising in them had been under supervision by authority, but now it was possible to inspect the facilities provided and require them to be remedied if they fell short of what was desirable. In the same year midwifery training was extended to six months for qualified general nurses, and to 12 months for others. Another advance of 1926 was that the Midwives Institute awarded a Midwife Teacher's Diploma for the first time. By this year immense progress had been made. A somewhat chaotic series of arrangements early in the century had been organized into sensible ones inside 25 years. An excellent teaching system for midwives, in theory and practice, was in place under the supervision of well-trained teachers. In 1933 the Central Midwives Board took over the running of the courses, the regulations of, and the training for the Midwife Teacher's Diploma.

In 1929 several hospitals in the UK were taken over by Local Authorities. Maternity departments in many of them were founded as a back up service for the domiciliary one. Until then the tasks of the Local Supervising Authorities were mainly concerned with the domiciliary service. But the birth rate was falling and this prompted political anxieties about the future population. In 1927 the proportion of hospital confinements was 15 per cent of all births. By 1932 it had risen to 24 per cent, and in 1937 to almost 35 per cent. In 1952 64 per cent of women were delivered in hospital.

Women themselves increasingly came to want hospital care. It was a change in cultural attitudes. Even in the 1930s and 1940s the maternal mortality was in the region of 5 per 1,000 total births. Perhaps many women were vaguely aware of this and felt that they might have a better chance of survival in hospital rather than at home. It was only later that the psychological drawbacks of admission to hospital and consequent separation from the rest of the family came to be appreciated.

In domiciliary practice, as mentioned earlier, midwives were allowed to administer gas and air analgesia to women in labour, provided that they were trained in its use. Later they could use 'Trilene' for the relief of pain.

In 1936 a new Midwives Act consolidated previous Acts and established a full-time municipal midwifery service. Every childbearing woman in each Local Supervising Authority area had by statute to have provision made for her maternity care. Those who were not looked after in hospitals came under the care of midwives paid by the Local Authority. They conducted antenatal clinics, delivered patients at home, in hospitals or maternity homes, and visited them at home in the puerperium. There were still private midwives but they too came under the control of the Local Authority Midwifery Supervisor, who in turn was accountable to the council's Medical Officer of Health.

In 1945 the Rushcliffe Committee recommended that no midwife should annually attend more than 65 cases of labour in domiciliary practice. This was a sensible recommendation and probably improved the service by making sure that midwives did not spread their work too thinly in the search for financial reward in private practice.

In 1947 the last of the untrained *bona fide* midwives left the Roll. Thereafter only those who had been properly trained and examined in accordance with the regulations of the Central Midwives Board could have their names on the Roll. Only they, and doctors, could then give maternity care.

In 1948 the National Health Service in the UK began. Under the Act of 1946 midwives had their professional position within it, both in hospital and domiciliary practice, firmly established. Moreover general practitioners attending maternity cases could only be paid out of public funds if their names were on a special obstetric list. Entry to that list, held by the Local Authority, was only allowed to those who had had approved postgraduate training in obstetrics. In effect this meant that if a midwife called in a general practitioner to help her in the management of a case, then she could be reasonably certain that he had at least some suitable knowledge and expertise. It had not always been so. Yet it still remained possible for general practitioners without much experience to undertake private practice in obstetrics. In hospitals, maternity care was in the hands of consultant obstetricians with a team of junior doctors, supporting the care given by midwives.

Midwifery practice was constrained by the Central Midwives Board in their promulgation of a booklet of *Midwives Rules.* These laid down, perhaps rather too rigidly at first, the conditions in which medical aid had to be called in. The Rules had to be strictly adhered to on pain of disciplinary action by the Authority and/or the Board, if they were not complied with. In 1947 the Rules were somewhat relaxed to allow midwives more personal initiative in their management of childbearing women. And in 1950 they were allowed to administer pethidine to women in labour without the necessity of consulting a doctor beforehand. Several other drugs have now been added to the list of those that may be prescribed and given. These changes rightly emphasized that midwives are independent practitioners within the limits laid down by the Central Midwives Board. They then became recognized as being the best persons to help women in the management of normal pregnancy, labour and the puerperium, as well as the care of the normal newborn. They were taught to recognize abnormalities in any of these phases and in both of their patients. When such abnormalities occurred or seemed to occur it was their duty to call in medical help.

Doctors

By a previous Medical Act it had been decreed that all undergraduate medical students had to have had experience of midwifery and the care of babies at the time of qualifying. This regulation had some success in improving the care of childbearing women. The training was still somewhat perfunctory, but it was better than doctors having no experience of midwifery at all. By far the greatest amount of midwifery care was in the hands of midwives and general practitioners in the decades around 1900. Their patients were delivered at home or in nursing homes with maternity facilities, which could vary greatly.

Prior to this doctors who wished to learn about midwifery sought out teachers, such as Smellie, Denman, Leake and many others in London, and there were several in Edinburgh and Dublin. In those two cities Chairs of Midwifery were established in the 18th century. One was founded in London in 1828 at University College and another in 1831 at King's College.

Even before the requirement of the General Medical Council that all should have studied midwifery before qualifying, both Cambridge and London Universities in 1841 required students in their final examinations to have knowledge of midwifery. By 1859 Cambridge insisted on students producing certificates of attendance on courses in 'Obstetric Medicine' before they were allowed to sit. Despite these moves, education in midwifery was sporadic, often non-existent, until the Medical Act of 1886.

In 1888 the General Medical Council decreed that every student should spend three months in a lying-in hospital and personally conduct 12 deliveries, three of which had to be under the supervision of a duly qualified practitioner. In 1895 and 1900 the British Medical Association, a non-statutory body, yet politically and educationally powerful, recommended to the General Medical Council that it should increase the amount of undergraduate time spent in studying midwifery. The BMA was representative particularly of general practitioners, and it was they who carried the major burden of maternity medical care at the time.

By 1922 the General Medical Council called for systematic instruction in midwifery, gynaecology and infant hygiene. It was to be in the basic principles, clinical instruction and attendance on practice for six months. There had to be practical hospital instruction in antenatal, intranatal, postnatal and puerperal care, together with infant care for a total of six months, two of which had to be spent in the lying-in hospital or wards, during which time 12 deliveries were to be personally conducted under senior supervision.

Increasingly during the first half of the 20th century maternity care shifted towards hospitals. In them were more and more specialists. There had been a few specializing in midwifery since the earliest times, from the days of the man-midwives and before that. Probable factors in later specialization were the founding of lying-in hospitals and wards, the introduction of the obstetric forceps and other necessary obstetric operations, aided by the use of anaesthesia. Gynaecology, which was allied with obstetrics, became a largely surgical specialty needing hospital facilities. Yet the way was not always smooth for obstetricians. For instance Charles James Cullingworth was appointed as an Obstetric Physician at St Thomas's Hospital, London, from his post in Manchester. At first he was not allowed to breach the peritoneum surgically. If he required a caesarean section to be done on one of his patients he had to request a general surgeon to perform the operation. Soon, however, this ridiculous restriction was withdrawn.

The attitudes of the general medical establishment towards obstetrics and gynaecology and their practitioners made them begin attempts to break away from the mainstreams of medicine and surgery. Obstetric and gynaecological societies were founded in Ireland in 1838 and the following year there was one in Edinburgh under the chairmanship of James Young Simpson. Similar societies began in the North of England and in the Midlands. In 1921 all came together in the first British Congress of Obstetrics and Gynaecology.

Out of this Congress and the powerful Gynaecological Visiting Society, which had been called into being by Blair Bell of Liverpool in 1911 – the first of its kind in the world – there came the College of Obstetricians and Gynaecologists. It was the first College to break away from the previously all-powerful Colleges of Surgeons and Physicians, by whom it was greatly resisted. The Royal College of Obstetricians and Gynaecologists received its charter in 1929. It was especially remarkable in that its writ ran throughout the whole British Empire of the time.

The RCOG quickly established its Membership by examination. This formalized and professionalized the specialty of Obstetrics and Gynaecology. The College laid down the curriculum to be followed by aspiring specialists, its length of time, the places in which education and training could be pursued under supervision, and it conducted a searching examination, which was written, clinical and oral. A book of case histories, with commentaries upon them, both in obstetrics and in gynaecology had to be submitted to be examined, before entry to the more formal examination was allowed. It can be seen that those who became Members were well-educated and well trained in their subjects. The examinations have changed in format over the years but the essentials remain the same. The diploma of MRCOG became the *sine qua non* to become a consultant in the National Health Service hospitals. More senior Members were elected to the Fellowship.

Later still the Royal College introduced a Diploma of Obstetrics to be awarded after appropriate posts in hospital and the passing of clinical, oral and written examinations. It was designed to be suitable for general practitioners, and showing that they had knowledge and competence beyond that required of the ordinary graduate in medicine. Those who obtained the D(Obst.) RCOG were able to perform the minor operations of obstetrics, including forceps deliveries, but were not usually with sufficient expertise and experience to perform caesarean sections. These educational moves for midwives, general practitioners and specialists may not have been of apparent significance for childbearing women but they undoubtedly improved the quality of the services rendered to them. All aspects of maternity became safer and physical care, especially of the serious emergencies improved almost beyond recognition as compared with previous epochs, because of educated and trained professionals.

Along with this progress in education and training came the development of specialist journals both for midwives and doctors. These aided the revision of knowledge and the dissemination of new knowledge. There had been the local societies and clubs which had often published their proceedings. Now, however, the community of obstetrics and midwifery became national and international. Several of the general journals devoted space to obstetric and gynaecological matters. Such were the *Edinburgh Medical and Surgical Journal* founded in 1905; the *Lancet* of 1823; the *British Medical Journal* of 1840 and many others. An interesting experiment of 1873 was the founding of the *Obstetrical Journal of Great Britain and Ireland*, which always contained an American supplement. It shows how international the subjects had become, though it only lasted for seven years. But the general journals were not enough. In 1902 the *Journal of Obstetrics and Gynaecology of the British Empire* began. It later became the *Journal of Obstetrics and Gynaecology of the British Commonwealth*, and later still the *British Journal of Obstetrics and Gynaecology*. Of course, similar specialist journals proliferated all over the world in America and the Antipodes especially.

Basic education and training followed by postgraduate and continuing education are now the hallmarks of any progressive profession. They are exemplified in the professions of midwifery and obstetrics, and they have raised the standards of service given to individual patients. Much remains to be done. There are initiatives arising within the professions, and from the public and their elected representatives which constantly change the nature, purpose and philosophy of professional education, and how the professions should develop to serve their communities better.

A widely publicized snide remark is that all professions are a conspiracy against the public, whom they are supposed to serve. It is said that their organization is essentially for the protection of their members. That may be partly true but ignores the fact that proper professionalization is a protection for the public too. The relationships between the professional organizations of midwifery and obstetrics and the public they serve should be mutually supportive and not antagonistic. Each depends on the other.

CHAPTER ELEVEN

Mortality Statistics

It is not intended to attempt to deal with these figures exhaustively. That is for treatises. Here the intention is to highlight something of the trends in recent years, with a view to showing their significance for the ways in which midwifery and obstetric practice have changed towards the end of the century.

Maternal mortality

This is defined as the number of maternal deaths per 1,000 total births, whether the babies are stillborn or alive. Twins and other multiple pregnancies are included so that the actual number of mothers is always slightly less than the number of 1,000. There have been attempts to measure the number of 'maternities' or, in effect, pregnancies. However, this has not been widely adopted. Most countries register births and deaths, so it is on these that international comparisons are based.

In England and Wales the Ministry of Health in 1928 instituted detailed investigations into the numbers and causes of maternal deaths. With some temporal gaps they have continued ever since. Since 1952 they have been a regular feature in obstetric practice. There have been similar investigations in Scotland and Northern Ireland, i.e. all parts of the United Kingdom. The figures used here are for England and Wales. For present purposes they are reasonably representative of most developed countries in the western world, though there are sometimes significant differences between them.

The Confidential Enquiries into Maternal Deaths cover periods of three years at a time. When a maternal death occurs the local Registrar of Births and Deaths notifies an appointed senior obstetrician. He or she is usually from a nearby teaching hospital. He or she consults with all those concerned with the particular death and asks for a special form to be filled in about it. On receipt of that form he or she can ask for further information from all people concerned. The attempt is made to determine just why the woman died, especially in the light of current acceptable practice. It is in no sense an attempt to apportion blame, and for this reason it is entirely confidential. Its intention is to collect and collate information. The standard of judgement about the management of the case is not that of the supposed very best practice, but rather of what might reasonably have been expected from all the professionals at all levels in the circumstances of the disaster. An attempt is made to decide whether, if reasonable, acceptable, care had been exercised, the death might have been avoided. This is not to say that the death could have been avoided, but might have been avoided. This concept of possible 'avoidable' deaths is at the heart of the Enquiry, pinpointing possible errors of clinical judgment and management, so that publicizing them may be a warning to others of the many dangers to childbearing women which can be minimised by good clinical care. When the regional investigator has finished, the report is sent to national assessors. They too can ask for further information if they believe that to be necessary and helpful in reaching a judgement. The results are published every three years for England and Wales. There is no way in which individual cases or professionals can be identified from the Reports. All professionals cooperate in the enquiry voluntarily. Yet in 1952–54 the response rate was 70 per cent and it has increased subsequently. The Reports, however, are therefore not based on all maternal deaths. The numbers of those are only obtainable from the Registrar General's tables, but these have not been examined in the same clinically thorough way as those of the Reports. The maternal mortality figures speak for themselves.

Table 11.1: Maternal mortality statistics 1928–1991

Years	Total Births	Maternal Deaths	Rate per 1,000
1928–30	> 2 million	7,561	3.78
1948–50	> 2.25 million	2,158	0.95
1958–60	2,322,229	928	0.40
1981–91	7,351,145	462	0.06

Maternal deaths fell to 1.6 per cent of their former value over about 60 years. (The above figures exclude deaths from abortion.) The causes of death were, as they always have been, pre-eclampsia/eclampsia, haemorrhages both antepartum and postpartum, pulmonary embolism, abortion, cardiac disease, caesarean section and anaesthesia. These are roughly in the order of numerical precedence, which has changed only slightly from triennium to triennium. Infection as a cause of death fell to very low levels after the introduction of chemotherapy and antibiotics. The following table is derived from one published by the Registrar-General.

Table 11.2: Decennial maternal mortality averages for England and Wales (per 1,000 live births)

Years	Puerperal	Sepsis	Others
1847–1854	5.4	1.8	3.6
1855–1864	4.7	1.6	3.1
1865–1874	5.0	1.9	3.1
1875–1884	4.6	2.3	2.3
1885–1894	5.1	2.6	2.4
1895–1904	4.6	2.1	2.5
1905–1914	3.9	1.6	2.2
1915–1924	3.9	1.5	2.4
1925–1934	4.3	1.7	2.6
1935–1944	2.9	0.8	2.1
1945–1950	1.2	0.17	1.07
1950	0.89	0.19	0.07
1952–1972	0.29		

Between 1855 and 1934 the total number of deaths for each ten-year period varied between 27,000 and 45,000. Each year therefore, between 3,000 and 4,000 women died as a result of childbirth. There is a dramatic decrease in the numbers of deaths caused by puerperal sepsis from 1935 onwards. Sulphonamides were introduced in 1936, and penicillin became widely available from about 1943 and after. Their use shows just how valuable they were in coping with puerperal infections. There were 11 deaths from puerperal sepsis in 1973–75 out of 1,940,689 births, c. 5.7 per million

During the triennium 1952–54 there were 246 deaths from pre-eclampsia/eclampsia in which 52 per cent had 'avoidable' factors in the strict sense accorded to that term (*vide supra*). There were 220 deaths from haemorrhages, and 64 per cent of these were thought to be 'avoidable'. Of the 220 deaths 53 were due to transfer from home to hospital of the patient in the third stage of labour with the placenta still retained within the uterus. This finding led to the founding of many more Flying Squads, and is an example of the value of the collection of these figures in causing change to safer practices.

Flying Squads consist of a midwife, an obstetrician, an anaesthetist, all in an ambulance and with equipment, especially blood, with blood transfusion and infant resuscitation apparatus, anaesthetic machine and obstetric implements, and a variety of drugs. Such a team is capable of dealing with most, if not all obstetric emergencies, short of caesarean section. Even that is possible in some dire circumstances. However the intention was to do the minimum possible for the safety of the patient prior to her transfer to hospital, but that included manual removal of the placenta under anaesthesia in the home. By 1955–57 the number of deaths from haemorrhage had fallen to 138, of which 24 were due to haemorrhage with a retained placenta. The mortality from that cause had been more than halved. It was not entirely due to the Flying Squads, but also due to increased awareness of the dangers from those practising domiciliary midwifery, so that patients were transferred earlier to hospital. The Reports had enormous educational value for the professionals.

From 1952 to 1960 the triennial Reports showed a decline in deaths from pre-eclampsia/eclampsia, from haemorrhages, from abortions, from cardiac disease and from caesarean section. There was little change in the deaths from pulmonary embolism. This shows increasing competence of professionals and their awareness of major obstetric problems and how they should be dealt with. Deaths directly due to pregnancy or childbirth numbered 472 during 1952–54. In 1973–75 the number was 140 over three years out of roughly the same number of births, c. 2 million. This was a vast change from the deaths of 3,000 to 4,000 per year earlier in the 20th century.

In 1950 61.2 percent of all births were in National Health Service hospitals. It rose to 64.6 per cent in 1957, and further still later. Among the one-third booked for delivery at home there is no doubt that many of them should not have been. Those were the ones at high-risk which had not been recognized. The high-risk mothers began to be defined. They were those who had had pre-eclampsia in a previous pregnancy; had bled during the present pregnancy; had previously had a stillbirth, a difficult forceps or other type of delivery or a caesarean section; or who had intercurrent disease, especially diabetes, hypertension, or renal disease. It is astonishing that some of these high-risks were frequently ignored by the domiciliary services and to a lesser extent by the hospital ones, thereby unnecessarily endangering the mother. The Reports are full of cases where although the blood pressure was recorded as high in pregnancy no action was taken until disaster struck. There are also examples of not recognizing the seriousness of any vaginal bleeding in pregnancy; of rupture of the uterus after a previous caesarean section; of futile attempts to deliver the placenta; and of bungled forceps deliveries. The publicity about all these did begin to direct the behaviour of professionals into safer channels.

The 1958–60 Report detailed the responsibility for 'avoidable' factors in the deaths. They were:

- the consultant or hospital staff in 85 cases;
- the general practitioner in 136 cases;
- the Local Authority Medical Officer in 12 cases;
- the midwife in 19 cases;
- the patient or a relative in 91 cases;
- others in 4 cases.

These figures firmly showed where education was most needed – mainly for doctors and patients. Midwives as a group were largely exonerated in these still alarming statistics. It was something of a surprise to find patients and their relatives as responsible in some cases. Regrettably this was through ignorance and sometimes wilful disregard of advice they had been given. But that shows a degree of mistrust and lack of communication between patients and their professional attendants which should not have arisen.

Despite this, just over 999 women out of every 1,000 survived their pregnancies, labours and puerperia in the 1950s. Even mothers undergoing caesarean section had a 1 in 500 chance of survival. It was even better if the operation were done electively rather than as an emergency. This low mortality was just as well since caesarean section was increasingly performed. From 1957 to 1960 the rate was 3.8–4.5 per cent of all births. In 1954 the rate in teaching hospitals was 7.4 per cent and 3.9 per cent in non-teaching hospitals. It was said that the difference was because the teaching hospitals took many of the more difficult cases, especially those with intercurrent diseases and potential obstetric problems. But there seemed to arise a culture among obstetricians of using caesarean section as a solution to many problems. It seems probable in retrospect that the pendulum swung too far in this direction, but even in 1993 there is a still higher caesarean section rate, approaching 10 per cent. In 1973-75 those deemed to be responsible for maternal deaths which might have been avoided were:

- the consultant or hospital staff in 112 cases;
- the general practitioner in 27 cases;
- the Local Authority Medical Officer in 1 case;
- the midwife in 5 cases;
- the patient or a relative in 48 cases;
- the anaesthetist in 32 cases;
- others in 5 cases.

Of the 230 cases, avoidable factors occurred in the antenatal period in 50 per cent, 29 per cent in labour and 21 per cent in the puerperium. Again this showed where more vigilance and more education was needed. General practitioners in this period conducted only very few deliveries as care tended to switch to hospitals. In their labour practice only one death occurred. Yet 26 deaths occurred in patients under their care and it was thought that these might have been avoided. The avoidable deaths in hospital are partly explicable by the great increase in hospital maternity care at this time. Among the deaths were some due to cardiac disease, rare hypertension (phaeochromocytoma), cancers, suicide, road accidents and several others. Childbearing women are as prone to intercurrent diseases and accidents as are the non-pregnant. Noteworthy was the appearance of anaesthesia as a cause of death. It showed the need for better training of anaesthetists deputed to help in operative deliveries, and for a better understanding by anaesthetists of the special dangers of obstetric anaesthesia. They needed to be specialists.

One interesting fact came out of these Reports, and later investigations of Perinatal Mortality. It was that there were different mortality rates in different parts of the country. The reasons were much investigated and several conclusions drawn. Very generally for present purposes, and therefore to some extent inaccurately, there was a gradient with results being the worst in the north and gradually improving towards the south-east. There was a similar gradient from west to east, that is from Wales and Cornwall to East Anglia and the London area. The differences were not entirely due to the quality and quantity of the services provided. There were more hospitals and maternity beds in the south-east in proportion to the population, and a greater proportion of deliveries were conducted in hospital. However, Scotland was just as well provided with hospital facilities and had a high ratio of consultants to numbers of births.

It was Professors Dugald Baird of Aberdeen and Will Nixon of London in the 1950s who first drew attention to the importance of socio-economic factors in midwifery practice. Their studies were based on the Social Classes as defined for statistical purposes by the Registrar-General. There was no political purpose in this classification. It was to gain insight into the nature of society and how different factors might affect its functioning. The five Social Classes are:

I   Managerial and professional;
II   Supervisory;
III   Skilled workers, e.g. plumbers, carpenters etc.;
IV   Semi-skilled workers, e.g. factory hands;
V   Unskilled, e.g. labourers, kitchen hands.

It will be realized that these are roughly in descending order of income, though, for instance, there are many artisans who earn more than some professionals. Yet there is more to it than income. There is a descending order of education and training. The sorts of houses and neighbourhoods in which these various groups live, their leisure activities, the schools their children attend, the foods they eat, the newspapers they read, the television programmes they watch, are all different statistically as even the most superficial amateur observation shows. These are not value judgments; they are observations of differences. The Social Classes each develop their own forms of culture, and attitudes based upon them, not least to childbirth and all its problems.

Maternal mortality, excluding abortions, fell to very low levels. It was down to 0.54 per 1,000 in 1952. It was 0.11 per 1,000 births, less than 1 in over 9,000 births, in 1975, and had been in that region for about five years. The Maternity Mortality in 1993 for the whole United Kingdom is about 7 per 100,000 births. It became a relatively poor measure of obstetric results. The deaths were important in themselves, of course, but here the intention was statistical. Nevertheless behind the statistics are the sum of many interacting factors of thousands of individuals. Among them are the women themselves and their families and their differing cultural attitudes and values, the pressure groups serving the interests of women and the professional bodies with their cultural attitudes and practices. The midwives, general practitioners, consultants and managers too have their input into the what they conceive to be the social, psychological and physical matters of importance.

From the purely professional point of view it is apparent that at least the physical care of childbearing women improved rapidly around the middle years of the 20th century. There were many fewer deaths of women and their babies than there had ever been before. It is these facts, demonstrably shown by the statistics, that were the basis from which new initiatives in all phases of childbearing became possible. These initiatives became directed especially to more intensive care of fetuses and babies and to the pyschology of women before conception and during pregnancy, labour, the puerperium and after. It is only when the destruction and mayhem of all these have been brought almost fully under control that attention can be paid to other factors, especially of psychology. It has been crudely yet truly said that the dead have no psychology. Only when physical death is prevented can psychology receive the importance it deserves and has always deserved.

Perinatal mortality

Attention turned to the newer concept of Perinatal Mortality Rate (PMR). This is the number of stillbirths and neonatal deaths in the first week of life, related to 1,000 births. This was a better measure of the outcome of obstetric care than stillbirths and neonatal deaths in the first month of life which had been recorded previously. It is obvious enough that stillbirths are due to some catastrophe of pregnancy or labour. But it began to be realized that factors operating while the fetus was in utero might affect its survival over the first few days after it was born. The fact of birth was not the natural cut-off point that it had seemed to be. Pregnancy, labour and the puerperium are a continuum. There are no definite breaks in the processes except those we choose to put there, in this case for statistical purposes. Perinatal mortality was a better indicator of the events of pregnancy and labour as regards the baby than stillbirths and neonatal deaths.

In 1952 the Perinatal Mortality Rate was 37.5 per 1,000 total births. This means that about 1 in 26 babies died as a result of some obstetric accident. By 1975 the rate had fallen to 19.3, meaning that 1 in 51 babies so died. In 1981 it was 11.8 and in 1992 7.9 or 1 in 126 births. More had to be done but these figures do show a marked improvement over time. Something was happening, but it was not easy to be sure exactly what. There were many interacting factors, of which probably improved obstetric care was only one.

Further investigation showed that the outcome of childbearing as measured by perinatal mortality depended to a great statistical extent on the age of the mother, her height, parity and her Social Class. Very young and older mothers had worse results than those from about 22 to 35 years of age. Taller women, those over about 5' 2" (157.5 cm) in height, had better results than those who were smaller. Women having their first babies had a worse outcome than those having second and third babies. Yet those having a fourth baby had about the same perinatal mortalities as those having a first one. Later babies after the fourth had a worse statistical prognosis. Social Class I women had statistically better perinatal mortalities than all other Classes. There was a gradient of worsening results from Social Class I through all the others to Social Class V. Those in the higher Social Classes tended to be taller, control their childbearing by contraception, and so have their babies at more suitable ages for the reduction of perinatal mortality.

It became obvious that virtually everything favoured the higher Social Classes. They were better educated in childhood, better nourished and so grew taller, than their counterparts in the lower Classes. It seemed likely that taller women nourished their own babies better than the smaller ones, and in general this appears to be true. Taller women of higher Social Class have fewer small babies, whether those are born prematurely or are classed as small-for-dates.

Over the generations the poorer people did become better educated and better nourished. They did grow taller and heavier. Yet as they did so those of the upper Social Classes also improved on their education and heights. So even though results for poorer people improved they did not catch up with those of the upper Classes, and remained, as it were, always a generation behind. These social factors were reinforced to some extent by biological ones. It was shown that taller women in the lower Social Classes tended to move up a Class on marriage, while those who were short in the higher Classes tended to move down a Class on marriage. Therefore the upper classes were recruiting better reproducers from those who were less well endowed as a Class than themselves.

Better nutrition in childhood and better education tend to lead to higher intelligence quotients, as measured by the usual tests. There is thus a correlation between intelligence and height. In general the taller the person the greater the intelligence statistically. It was shown that the proportion of Social Class I people in the population was about 20 per cent in the south-east of the country, round London, but was only about ten per cent in the north and in Scotland.

It began to appear that not only did the south-east have advantages of hospital beds and numbers of consultants, it also had intrinsically better 'material' to work with. So many of the patients were taller, heavier, of controlled parity at various ages, and better educated than those elsewhere. It must be emphasized again that this is only statistical and must not be applied literally to individuals. So the gradients in mortality running from north to south and from west to east were in large measure dependent upon socioeconomic and biological factors which produced a better, more successful, childbearing population in the south-east and East Anglia than elsewhere. Moreover these upper Class people were articulate and wielded political clout so that they demanded and received better facilities.

None of these socio-biological considerations should diminish the facts that obstetric and medical care had also made a contribution to the better results. It is obvious that they have had an effect which should neither be denied nor over-emphasized.

The causes of maternal deaths had been investigated for some time, to the relative neglect of stillbirths, neonatal and infant deaths. This reflected the general understanding that the mother was far more important than the baby, if their interests conflicted at any time in the childbearing process. With the safety of mothers from dying now more or less assured it was time to turn greater attention to the welfare of the fetus and newborn. Stillbirths were classified as being macerated or fresh. Those macerated, that is to some extent aseptically decomposed, had obviously died some little time before birth. The process of maceration takes at least a few days to develop. The probable cause of such a death was almost certainly some degree of failure of the placenta. Further thought and investigation about this suggested that there were four essential functions of the placenta – nutrition, excretion, respiration and hormone production. Failure of the placenta to support adequate nutrition results in babies being small for dates at birth. Excretion has turned out so far to be almost impossible to measure. The products of excretion are lost amid those of the mother. The endocrine function is mainly concerned with altering the physiology of the mother in ways of value to the growth and wellbeing of the fetus.

Deaths in utero are almost always due to lack of oxygen (asphyxia) supplied to the fetus through the placenta. This is called anoxaemia. The supply and excretion of all nutrients depend on:

1.   the maternal blood supply,
2.   the tissues of the placenta and their functions, and
3.   the fetal blood supply.

Attention was concentrated on the maternal blood supply. It was known to be diminished in cases of hypertension and pre-eclampsia, in both of which conditions the stillbirth rate was higher than average. But perhaps there were also cases where the maternal blood supply to the placenta was diminished without any overt signs in the mother. The efficiency of the fetal circulation was unknown and resisted attempts at direct measurement. Cases of fetal anaemia due to the erythroblastosis fetalis of Rhesus disease were known to cause death. Nevertheless there remained a large number of macerated stillbirths which were inexplicable by the knowledge of the time.

Fresh stillbirths are those where the baby dies as a result of factors operating during labour. They are more certainly attributable to acute anoxia or trauma sustained during birth. Obvious examples are where the umbilical cord prolapses and is trapped so that the fetal circulation is arrested. In prolonged labours the uterus contracts and slowly cuts off or diminishes the blood supply to the maternal side of the placenta. The separation of the placenta in accidental haemorrhage or placenta praevia cuts off maternal circulation completely. This is also especially likely to occur in breech delivery for the uterus is emptied of the baby's body so that the placenta separates from the uterine wall, while the baby's head may remain in the vagina where it may suffocate before it is able to breathe.

There is also the possibility of birth trauma, especially to the head, causing intracranial haemorrhage, which if severe enough causes death. This can occur where there is gross disproportion between the size of the head and the pelvis, in malpresentations, in difficult forceps deliveries and in breech deliveries. All may cause great compression of the head, which in the fetus is easily distorted and liable to tearing of structures within it and consequent bleeding within the substance of the brain.

In 1946 A. MacGregor of Edinburgh analysed by post-mortem the causes of death in 453 stillbirths and 618 neonatal deaths.

The results were:

Asphyxia	22 per cent
Birth injury	26 per cent
Infection	19 per cent
Malformations	14 per cent
Other causes	18 per cent

This shows that the major causes of death were asphyxia, injury and infection which caused 67 per cent of all deaths. The remedies lay in the hands of the doctors. Asphyxia, injury and infection during labour were all in essence preventable by good obstetric care. Even some of the factors operable in pregnancy might be controlled by effective antenatal treatment of hypertension, diabetes, renal disease and pre-eclampsia. Malformations in the circumstances of the time could not be prevented. That was a matter for later.

There was a massive Perinatal Mortality Survey in 1958. During one week all stillbirths, perinatal deaths, deaths in the first week as well as the first month of life were notified to a central register. During the following three months intensive investigation of deaths was carried out by post-mortem examinations. The detailed results are not of immediate importance here, though they were immensely valuable at the time and subsequently. They confirmed the essential results in the above table. The book was a mile post on the journey towards the goal of providing ever better obstetric and then paediatric care. In effect it defined the state of things as they then were and, just like the Confidential Maternal Mortality Reports before them, showed which problems needed attention. The message as in maternal mortality was the same. Unremitting care by all professionals was essential to attain to reduction of maternal and perinatal deaths. If all professionals put into practice what was already known then all women and their babies would be safer. New research would undoubtedly come along but the need was to apply with increasing vigilance the knowledge already gained.

Doctors and midwives had to be better trained and educated and apply what they had learned conscientiously and with unflagging vigour and attention to duty.

CHAPTER TWELVE

Trends After 1950

There can be no detailed account of midwifery and obstetrics which will do other than summary justice to the ways in which they have changed during this recent period. So many of the problems which had bedevilled childbearing and childbirth for centuries were almost suddenly solved, or so it seemed. The physical care of women in pregnancy, labour and the puerperium was virtually codified and adopted in every advanced country. It had become a matter of unremitting routine, and for many women that was exactly its fault and a main source of justified criticism. The more perceptive of them felt as if they were being dealt with like objects on a factory assembly line. A certain insensitiveness seemed to creep into the minds of the professionals, as they went about their work, so that they appeared to their patients to be uncaring and mechanistic. The professionals concentrated on producing live and healthy babies and mothers at the end of the childbearing process. In view of what had gone before in earlier times it is not perhaps surprising that this was their main aim and objective. The deaths and mayhem of earlier times were ever present in their minds, and above all they had to be prevented. It took time for it to be recognised that a watershed in professional management had been reached.

New directions were called for, building on the success of physical care and its outcomes, especially for the mother. She was no longer normally at serious risk of death or incapacitating prolonged illness as a result of childbirth. It was still otherwise for the baby. There were too many perinatal deaths (stillbirths and first-week deaths), and even deaths in the first month of life. Attention was therefore turned much more towards the baby's welfare, both in utero and immediately after birth. The baby was seen to be at least of equal importance with the mother, perhaps for the first time in history. Much work was done in attempting to understand the intrauterine environment. This demanded scientific techniques of investigation beyond the relatively simple clinical ones of earlier midwifery and obstetrics. Scientific monitoring in pregnancy and labour became *de rigeur*, at first in advanced units and later in virtually all of them, as the techniques were simplified and made more easily available. The needs of the baby up to the time of birth were increasingly understood and acted upon. The needs of the baby after birth were realized to be beyond the haphazard care and competence of the average obstetrician and ordinary midwives, when there was trouble. So arose the speciality of neonatal paediatrics.

It was an advance in care when paediatricians first came to be introduced on a regular basis into the labour wards for babies thought to be at risk. There they could undertake resuscitation of the newborn and deal with the emergencies arising. A little later it was recognized that even they had to learn special techniques of caring for the neonate, which were different from those needed for the care of older children. A little later still the neonatal paediatricians needed to work in a team with paediatric surgeons, and the especially important trained neonatal intensive care nurses and midwives. The previously amateur care of the newborn was properly handed over to professionals. Paediatricians became part of the labour ward team. The same specialization and professionalization came about in anaesthesia too. Obstetricians had, in not too distant times, turned their hands to 'rag and bottle' anaesthesia, and even sometimes caudal anaesthesia. But this was no longer enough. General anaesthetists had taken over for caesarean sections, for this was seen as a major operation comparable with many others. But even this was not enough for it was slowly appreciated that anaesthesia for pregnant women presented special problems and dangers, as the Confidential Enquiries into Maternal Deaths had vividly shown, for there were many avoidable deaths attributed to anaesthesia. Moreover anaesthesia, indifferently practised, could be deleterious for the baby as well. The only proper response was to develop obstetric anaesthesia as a speciality, just as had been the case in neurosurgery, cardiac and chest surgery. Any general anaesthesia, for whatever even supposedly minor purpose, had to be in the hands of experts. Only local anaesthesia, that is perineal infiltration or pudendal block, remained properly in the hands of obstetricians.

Radiology was less used in pregnancy because Alice Stewart of Oxford had shown that irradiation of the embryo and to a lesser extent of the fetus led to an increased risk of leukaemia later in the life of the child. Yet there was some resurgence in radiologists' activities in obstetrics with the advent of ultrasound as a diagnostic tool, introduced by Professor Ian Donald (1910–1982) of Glasgow. This non-invasive harmless technique revolutionized much of obstetrics. It came into routine use in many clinics for estimating the size of the fetus early and late in pregnancy so that maturity and retarded growth could be more exactly recognized than previously. Normal growth of the fetus is probably the best general estimate of a sustaining intrauterine environment. If the baby is growing well then the mother is providing the right environment and the placenta is working effectively in its respiratory, nutritive, excretory and endocrine functions. Ultrasound was used for locating the placenta too and for diagnosing some fetal abnormalities. It was in attempting to measure these vital functions of the feto-placental unit that there had to be recourse to scientific monitoring investigations. It is these, among many others, that have caused much public anxiety in the mid-1990s.

Pathological laboratories were increasingly used. There was a place for all four disciplines of haematology, microbiology, chemical pathology and morbid anatomy. Every woman needed blood investigations, and bacteriology when there were vaginal or urinary infections. Biochemical investigations were required for hormonal assays and abnormal blood chemistry. Morbid anatomical investigations help with understanding diseases of the placenta and those of stillbirths and neonatal deaths. For any woman suspected of having cardiac, respiratory, renal, thyroid disease or diabetes, or indeed any illness, physicians had to be consulted. Care was often shared between them and obstetricians.

Teamwork among a variety of specialist professionals was needed for the best practice and the best results for mothers and their babies. No one person, nor even two or three, is now capable or competent enough in all the disciplines needed to deliver proper care to pregnant, labouring and puerperal women. The care of neonates too demands the combined and coordinated efforts of a large team. That many members of the team function behind the scenes and are not always centre stage should not be lost sight of. They are important and necessary. Their contributions to women's welfare should not be forgotten nor minimized. The problem for a childbearing woman is that she needs to relate psychologically to only one or two professional persons. The whole team is too discrete to be of value to her in this personal context. Inevitably it is the midwife and obstetrician who, to her, must be seen as the leaders and coordinators of the team which is acting on her behalf. It is unfortunate that to many women these two groups seem often to have failed in their tasks of communicating fully with their charges. They have sometimes seemed abrupt, off-hand, even unkind, largely because of ignorance of their patients' needs for understanding, and because even if they did have knowledge of patient anxieties they did not know how to alleviate them. In the later decades of the century this neglect of pyschological care is slowly changing and improving, mainly because of the activities of women's pressure groups, which have made great headway in voicing their concerns and having them heeded by the professionals.

Antenatal care

Antenatal care flourished in hospitals, Local Authority Clinics, midwives' clinics and doctors' surgeries during this period. Every woman became aware of the need to go to a doctor or clinic when she knew or thought she was pregnant. The philosophy of antenatal care was to discover any general bodily disorders and to treat them, and at the same time look out for more specific obstetric problems and those affecting or likely to affect the fetus. A medical and surgical history was taken to find out about pre-existing dieases, especially cardiac, respiratory, renal and endocrine ones such as diabetes. An obstetric history was recorded to show the details of previous babies, their ages, birth weights, anomalies, subsequent progress and whether born alive or dead, and the mode of delivery, e.g. by forceps or caesarean section. It was necessary to know too about previous infertility, miscarriages, premature births or any complications of pregnancy such as pre-eclampsia or antepartum bleeding, in attempting to be aware of and offset, if possible, any risks in the present pregnancy.

A general physical examination was made. While examining the chest the opportunity was taken to examine the breasts, and particularly note whether the nipples were flat, indrawn or protruding. If flat or indrawn the woman was often told to draw the nipple out with her finger and thumb. Some were given nipple shields to be worn under the bra, so that the nipple protruded through a hole. Probably these techniques were useless for the purpose for which they were intended, i.e. easy breastfeeding, by having the nipple stand out. There was some useful purpose, however, in cleaning the nipple regularly and rubbing in some simple ointment. This tended to prevent cracking of the nipple later, in the puerperium. There was a vogue for encouraging breastfeeding even in those who did not wish to do so. It coincided to some extent with the increased interest in the emotions experienced by childbearing women. It was felt that the bodily intimacies between mother and baby, inseparable from breastfeeding, established psychological bonds between them which were beneficial to both. This was an hypothesis difficult to prove yet it seemed sensible enough, but it was pursued by some with unnecessary fanaticism. There were many excellent mothers who felt emotionally and physically incapable of breastfeeding. Yet they were chivvied to do so and could be made to feel miserable and failures as mothers. It was yet another demonstration of how fashions and cultures change in reproductive practices. Some doctors, midwives, articulate busybodies and many journalists cotton on to an idea, shout it from the housetops, try to force it on to others, thinking they have discovered a universal truth. Individual variations from that truth are condemned, not appreciating the unpleasant effects of the condemnation on its recipients and forgetting that people do differ from one another and by being different they are not to be classed as sinners.

One clinical practice which was probably of value was that of expression of the breasts. The woman herself was to hold a breast at its base between both hands and then gently massage the breast towards the nipple. At the end of pregnancy this often expelled dried plugs of milk (or colostrum) from the ducts, so preventing blockage. Moreover it was a useful technique in the puerperium if and when the breasts overfilled and the baby was not fully removing the milk by suckling. The excess of milk could then sometimes be expressed from the breast to give relief from discomfort and pain.

The normal thyroid gland enlarges in pregnancy but evidences of hyperthyroidism were looked for in case the disorder needed treatment.

Cardiac murmurs were especially noted. Cardiac disease had become a numerically important cause of maternal death as other more definitely obstetric causes came to be controlled. Doubtful murmurs were elucidated by cardiac physicians and management then became a matter of cooperation and consultation between the obstetrician and the physician.

Respiratory disorders, particularly tuberculosis, were rarely picked up by clinical examination. Routine chest X-rays were the order of the day. Doubtful cases were referred to chest physicians, who, if possible, confirmed the diagnosis of tuberculosis, by bacteriological examination of the sputum or by laryngeal washings. Fortunately treatment had tended to move out of the sanatorium and thoracic surgical wards because chemotherapy with streptomycin, isoniazid and para-amino-salicylic acid (and later other drugs) had made prolonged in-patient treatment unnecessary. As pulmonary tuberculosis became rarer, because of effective treatment, routine chest X-rays were slowly abandoned. They had caused some anxiety since often the examination had been performed without adequate screening of the abdomen. The scatter of the rays was probably a danger to the embryo and fetus, even with the abdomen screened with lead, perhaps causing genetic changes which would express themselves later. Leukaemia had already been shown to be a consequence of indiscriminate obstetric radiology during pregnancy.

Abdominal palpation was a feature of every antenatal visit. After about 12 weeks of pregnancy the fundus of the uterus can be felt in the abdomen and the regularity of its growth over the months gave some indication that all was progressing normally. There came a vogue for measuring the height of the fundus above the symphysis pubis with a tape measure. Some used to record the abdominal girth at the umbilicus. The accuracy and value of these measurements were doubtful, and were superseded by more scientific monitoring of the function of the feto-placental unit. Clinical attempts to judge the size of the fetus by palpation near term were proven to be notoriously inaccurate despite some claims to the contrary.

Vaginal examinations were routinely performed at an early visit to the clinic, no longer so much for estimating the size of the bony pelvis, but rather for discovering any abnormalities of the soft parts of the pelvis. They are rare yet important for there may be no other way to diagnose them unless it be by ultrasound, which in the early part of this period was not widely available. Towards term abdominal palpation determined the lie, presentation and position of the baby. The degree of engagement of the head in the pelvis and its flexion was gauged. The fetal heart was listened to and a guess at the baby's weight was made. Transverse lies were corrected by external version, but they often recurred. If external version seemed likely to be easy and to succeed it was used in breech presentations. Otherwise breech presentations and transverse lies were left to be dealt with later.

Blood pressure was recorded at every visit to the antenatal clinic. The major sign of pre-eclampsia is raised blood pressure; above 140 mmHg systolic and 90 mmHg diastolic were the generally agreed figures. There are no symptoms in the early stages. Urine was tested for protein and sugar at every visit. Proteinuria is another sign of pre-eclampsia. Glycosuria may be indicative of diabetes, and it may begin for the first time in pregnancy. It can be a very serious complication of pregnancy, especially affecting the baby though there are other more benign forms of glycosuria.

Oedema (swelling due to fluid) was looked for over the lower shin bones and to a lesser extent over the sacrum, by pressing the tissues with a finger to see if there was any continuing indentation where fluid had been forced away from the site. Undue swelling is another sign of pre-eclampsia. This disorder may affect as many as 15 per cent of women in a first pregnancy. If it occurs then, it is even more likely to occur in subsequent pregnancies. If pre-eclampsia is allowed to progress its effects can be devastating, even as far as death of both baby and mother. Weighing at every visit was carried out. Undue weight gain of more than about 1lb (0.5kg) per week in the later weeks of pregnancy gave a hint of the possibility of fluid retention, which is sometimes associated with pre-eclampsia.

In the laboratory the blood group, Rhesus type and haemoglobin levels were determined. A blood transfusion may be needed suddenly in pregnancy or in labour. Knowing the blood group helped in quicker cross-matching of the blood to be given. Anaemia is extremely common in pregnancy and needs to be diagnosed. It is usually due to shortage of iron, but can be due to lack of folic acid. In most clinics it became routine to give all pregnant women both iron and folic acid as a preventive measure. The Rhesus factor determination was essential for the proper care of the fetus and the prevention, or rather more rarely the treatment in utero of the various forms of erythroblastosis fetalis.

Other blood tests were performed to diagnose previous syphilis or gonorrhoea. The Wassermann Reaction, and later other tests, were reasonable indicators of syphilis having been contracted in the past. The tests for gonorrhoea were very much less reliable. Because of the serious effects for the baby of the mother contracting German measles in pregnancy, tests were performed for the presence of rubella antibodies in the blood. Later there came immunization programmes where rubella vaccine was given to all girls aged about 12–15. This has been a most valuable preventive measure, almost eliminating congenital defects of the baby due to rubella.

More and more tests on the blood kept coming into practice. Alpha-fetoprotein estimations in patients thought to be at risk of having babies with open lesions of the central nervous system (spina bifida and anencephaly) showed many of them to have excessive quantities of the protein in the blood. Tests were also more frequently carried out by analysis of liquor amnii withdrawn from the uterus by a long needle and syringe passed through the abdominal and uterine walls. Cells showed the sex of the fetus. Some familial genetic diseases affect only one sex. In certain cases the parents may wish to have an abortion of those fetuses at special risk. Decision of course needed help from a geneticist. This is yet another example of the need for teamwork.

The foregoing is not intended to be a full description of antenatal care during this period, but rather to give a flavour of how it had changed since the first half of the century. It was more scientific and intensive, for women were seen even in normal pregnancy monthly to the 32nd week, fortnightly to the 36th week and weekly thereafter till delivery. For many women it was a matter of teamwork between general practitioners, obstetricians, midwives, laboratories, radiologists and a variety of other specialists in medical disciplines. This change from the apparent omnicompetence of a single doctor or midwife was not widely appreciated or understood, nor is it still, either among professionals or their patients.

The change in emphasis towards the welfare of the baby was not fully appreciated at the time either. Small (under 5lbs or 2.5kg) babies had been known to be at special risk of disease and death shortly after birth. They were all classed as premature to begin with. Then it was realized that some were premature in the sense of being born some time before the usual 40 weeks of pregnancy. They were so classified if they were born before the 37th week. They were small because they had not spent sufficient time in utero. But there were others who were small-for-dates or light-for-dates. These were obviously those who had been malnourished in utero. There must in them have been some failure of the placenta to satisfy their needs for growing and maturing. This led to attempts to assess the functioning of what came to be known as the feto-placental unit.

The functions of the placenta are nutritional, respiratory, excretory and endocrine. The respiratory function is of supreme importance during labour. It is then that acute anoxia can kill the baby either just before or just after birth. But the possible chronic anoxia during pregnancy could not easily be recognized, except perhaps by some invasive technique to take blood from the fetus, and this could not at first be countenanced. Direct transfer of nutrients to the fetus could not be measured either for that too would have required both maternal and fetal blood sampling. But the growth of the baby is an expression of its nutritional state. It became more surely measurable only with the advent of ultrasound techniques.

Ultrasound can measure the size of the fetal head (by its bi-parietal diameter), its abdominal girth and its crown-rump length. Most of these were known from previous simple clinical observations of babies born at varying lengths of gestation. Graphs could be constructed using these and plotting them against the length of pregnancy. They became refined using data from wide use of ultrasound at different lengths of pregnancy. The emphasis was particularly on the bi-parietal diameter of the skull. If the growth in this over time was within normal limits by comparison with the standards previously determined then all was likely to be well. The growth of the rest of the body, and the total weight, could be assumed correctly to be normal also. This was a major advance. It became routine to carry out ultrasound investigation at about 16 weeks of pregnancy and then at about 32 weeks. On a graph these two measurements showed whether growth was within normal limits or falling behind what was to be expected. If growth was severely impaired, as shown by serial observations over time, it was essential to deliver and rescue the baby from a deteriorating nutritional environment.

Prior to this more or less direct measure of fetal growth it had been usual to estimate the function of the placenta by the use of endocrine assays, mainly at first in urine. It was realized that these estimates were only an indirect measure of the function of the placenta as regards nutrition of the fetus, but they were the best then available. They were valuable nevertheless, relative failure in endocrine function tending to parallel failure of the other functions.

Chorionic gonadotrophin in early pregnancy, well-known from pregnancy tests was widely used, supplemented by pregnanediol (the excretory product of progesterone) estimations. They could be helpful in the management of threatened abortions. Later in pregnancy oestriol (the excretory product of oestrogens) and pregnanediol were used. Then came Human Placental Lactogen (HPL). The power of the placenta to produce an immense variety of hormones and enzymes came to be appreciated. Various attempts were made to measure them as indicators of the functions of the feto-placental unit. Blood assays were increasingly used.

It will be seen that antenatal care was by no means the simple routine that it might have seemed to the casual observer. Problems for the woman and her baby might be picked up at the first visit, or they might develop at some later time. The midwife and obstetrician had to remain very alert to a variety of potentially damaging deviations from the normal. They were both expert in the management and understanding of more or less obstetrical difficulties, but there were many others which had to be recognized so that the help of experts in other fields could be called upon for consultation and assistance. This even extended to surgical help, for abdominal emergencies may arise in pregnancy, and towards the latter part of this period patients were seen who had had renal transplantations, and they needed special observation and care.

Treatments of many diseases incidental to pregnancy had to be chosen with care. Pregnancy can alter the reaction of patients to treatments. Some might cause uterine contractions and premature labour. There is the possible effect of treatment on the embryo and fetus to be considered also. Some drugs may cause congenital anomalies in the baby. This was vividly shown by the thalidomide tragedy and by the use of phenytoin in the treatment of epilepsy. These drugs cause gross abnormalities of development of the limbs. The management of thyroid disorders and diabetes may lead to problems in the baby too. No wonder that teamwork came to be necessary. In perhaps 10–20 per cent of women there arose problems not fully soluble by the midwifery team alone.

Since several of the medical, surgical and obstetric problems were complex there had to be increasing recourse to admission of patients to hospital. Of the total complement of beds in a maternity hospital or unit it was usual to set aside about 25 per cent of them for pregnant women. Those with diseases incidental to childbearing needed careful frequent monitoring of progress. So did those with pre-eclampsia, poor fetal growth and antepartum haemorrhages. An unstable lie of the fetus required admission to hospital near term so that when labour supervened it could be made longitudinal for safety. The contractions of the uterus then held the longitudinal lie obtained by external version. This avoided the dire consequences of neglected transverse lie in labour.

Antepartum haemorrhage
Placenta praevia

Any cases of painless bleeding, however slight, were looked upon as being likely to be due to placenta praevia. That demanded immediate admission to hospital, for experience showed that a few such cases could suddenly bleed profusely without warning and put the mother's and the baby's lives at serious risk. With the woman in hospital the worst effects of massive haemorrhage could be offset by early transfusion and rapid delivery by the most appropriate means, often caesarean section. But by contrast it had been shown that many patients with painless slight bleeding had no further problems either in pregnancy or labour. Several of them had only the most minor degree of placenta praevia and a few did not have the disorder at all. Some were found to have *marginal sinus rupture* when the delivered placenta was examined. Round the edge of the placenta there runs a sinus of blood. Its outer wall is a fairly thin membrane, which can be breached if slightly malformed or if it should become inflamed and weakened. Slight painless bleeding per vaginam may then occur. The symptom can occur in some lesions of the cervix, such as cancer or a benign polyp. These need treatment in their own right. It became important to recognize the various non-urgent haemorrhages so that women should not be kept in hospital, away from their families, for inordinately long periods of time quite unnecessarily. Everything depended on knowing exactly where the placenta was located in the uterus. Clinically this was not determinable, except under general anaesthesia, when digital vaginal examination might or might not show the placenta to be partially or wholly in the lower uterine segment.

Amniography, straight radiology of the abdomen, and cystography had had some limited success in showing the position of the placenta, but something more accurate was needed. Arteriography by the injection of radio-opaque substances had come to be used safely in many medical and surgical conditions. It was imported into obstetric practice, injecting the dye into a femoral artery in the groin, the procedure being called retrograde femoral arteriography. It was excellent in showing up the arterial tree leading to the placenta, so was a better locator of the placenta than most other previous methods. Yet there was the danger of tearing the arterial wall with consequent serious local haemorrhage. The effects of the quite high radiation dose on the fetus also caused anxiety. The method was not used for long.

Another technique was to inject a radio-isotope and find by a radiation counter where it pooled in the vicinity of the uterus. The massive pool was, of course, the placental site.

All these earlier techniques were superseded by the use of ultrasound. Ultrasonic echoes reflect from the placenta, as well as the fetus, and they demonstrated its position. The technique was especially valuable, not only because it was accurate but also because it was and is non-invasive and causes no damage to either maternal or fetal tissues. It was also used for determination of the placental site before amniocentesis, that is when a needle is inserted into the liquor to withdraw a sample for analysis. If the needle is passed blindly into the liquor it may very well pass through the placenta. This may not be a cause of serious haemorrhage locally but fetal blood may be leaked into the maternal circulation. This can be a cause of antibody formation in the mother which is important in the genesis of Rhesus disease and therefore to be avoided. Knowing the site of the placenta the needle can be directed to avoid it.

When it seemed certain that there was not a placenta praevia the woman could often be discharged from hospital with safety. Those with definite placenta praevia had to undergo the treatment previously described. This was to keep the patient in bed with a view to minimizing the danger of further bleeding while the fetus grew on and matured. When thought to be mature and of adequate birth weight by clinical perception supported by ultrasound measurement of the bi-parietal diameter of the head, the woman was taken to the operating theatre with everything prepared for a caesarean section. This was preceded by a vaginal examination to make sure that the placenta could quite certainly be felt in the lower segment. Even ultrasound can occasionally mislead so it was wise to check the findings clinically. The examination included passing a finger through the cervix and into the lower uterine segment. It was a sensible rule that if the placenta could be felt at all then it was best to perform caesarean section for the sake of both mother and baby. The old grading system for placenta praevia was superseded as being unnecessary. When the placenta could not be felt the membranes were ruptured and a Syntocinon drip put up to send the woman into labour, which it was hoped and expected would be normal.

The waiting regime was, of course, interrupted at any time if massive bleeding occurred. Transfusion of blood was then essential prior to an emergency caesarean section. The baby might then be premature and require intensive neonatal paediatric care. But over the years the survival rate for such tiny babies improved beyond recognition as paediatricians, and especially the Special Care Baby nurses, became so expert in understanding and treating their tiny charges. Around the mid-century there was anxiety about the survival of any baby before the 37th week of pregnancy and weighing perhaps less than 5lb (2.5kg), and many succumbed. Gradually the loss of babies born before the 34th (c.2kg or less) and then the 32nd week was greatly reduced. This meant that obstetricians in consultation with neonatal paediatricians could undertake caesarean section, when necessary, earlier and earlier in pregnancy. Formerly a baby of 32–34 weeks maturity had poor chances of survival. By 1980 or so their chances in the Special care Nursery were very good.

The earlier history of this condition shows that the majority of women died if they had placenta praevia, and virtually all the babies perished too. Very slowly the safety of women was increasingly assured as a result of blood transfusion, general anaesthesia and less hazardous caesarean section. When that happened more attention could be paid to the fetus and neonate. This it received with magnificent results as compared with earlier times.

Abruptio placentae

This term replaced the older one of accidental haemorrhage. It came to be understood that abruptio was a distinct clinical entity, as placenta praevia was recognized to be. Apart from these two there was a miscellaneous collection of slighter antepartum bleeds, for example from marginal sinus rupture or very mild degrees of praevia, or rare cervical lesions.

The classical picture of abruptio is of severe sudden pain, followed by continuing unremitting pain caused by the tightly contracted uterus. The first pain is due to the separation of the placenta from the uterine wall. The patient is ashen and in agony, showing all the signs of internal bleeding, i.e. shock – with coldness, rapid pulse and lowered blood pressure. There can be many lesser forms of the disorder showing short lived more bearable pain and a tight uterus. After delivery the placenta then may show, in these lesser separations, the presence of an old or recent blood clot on its maternal surface. In all forms of abruption there is a slight loss of blood per vaginam.

Two wrong theories stood in the way of effective treatment for major abruption. The first was the belief that the condition was a complication of pre-eclampsia. In some cases just after the preliminary abruption the blood pressure is slightly raised above normal. It was therefore postulated, on virtually no evidence, that the blood pressure had been higher still just prior to the event. This meant that there was reluctance to transfuse blood in adequate quantities for fear of raising the blood pressure to its supposed former heights. In fact the blood pressure tends to drop in these cases as the blood is given, even when previously raised.

The explanation for these odd findings came from the early treatment of battle casualties. If these are reached quickly by paramedics the blood pressure is slightly raised despite large losses of blood. The reason is massive vascular contraction, raising peripheral resistance, which is the physiological response to haemorrhage. Blood pressure is the resultant of cardiac output and peripheral resistance. Later the blood volume falls so far that the spasm can no longer maintain the blood pressure. Patients suffering from abruptio placentae are exactly similar in their response to serious haemorrhage. The condition is so overwhelming that attendants arrive quickly on the scene, that is in the early phases of blood loss. The blood pressure is then slightly raised, though an hour or two later it usually falls to dangerous levels.

The second false theory was that the hard uterus was paralysed and would not begin to contract until some time had passed. This was based on the fact that many of these patients suffer from post-partum haemorrhage. The only known cause at the time was a relaxed, flaccid uterus which could not be made to contract and close off the blood vessels. In fact the cause of the post-partum haemorrhage in abruptio is lack of one or more clotting factors in the blood, mainly fibrinogen. The large quantities of blood shed internally from the vascular beds of the uterus and abdomen use up enormous quantities of all clotting factors. Slowly, as a result of this newer understanding and knowledge, it came to be realised that the uterus in abruptio was not paralysed but in a state of overall contraction, but without polarity such as occurs in labour when contractions start at the upper pole of the uterus and pass downwards ripple-like towards the cervix.

Once these two errors came to be slowly recognized the treatment became more rational. Pain had to be relieved with repeated opiate or pethidine injections. Blood transfusions had to be massive, giving two to three pints rapidly and then following up with more blood as the clinical state demanded. Overtransfusion was prevented sometimes by monitoring the venous pressure in the neck by a needle in the external jugular vein. The danger was most likely to be undertransfusion, and if the blood pressure remained low there was the possibility of pre-renal anuria resulting, because of inadequate perfusion of the kidneys. Such renal failure is a threat to life.

As soon as the clinical condition stabilized the membranes were ruptured to send the woman into labour. The cervix was always slightly dilated and taken up and the membranes bulged through it. These are both signs of high pressure within the uterus. Labour tended to follow and be quite short. Only rarely was a Syntocinon intravenous drip also required. Unfortunately the baby was almost invariably dead in the worst cases. This is not surprising for the whole placenta might be separated from the uterine wall, leaving the fetus without oxygen and a blood supply. In a few cases where the baby survived it was shown that if more than one-third of the placenta was separated the baby could not survive.

Only very rarely did there seem to be a case for caesarean section to be performed for the sake of the baby. In a few intances the fetal heart could be heard even after definitely diagnosed abruptio. Regrettably however the damage was already done to the fetus despite its struggles to live. All too often the baby died an hour or two after birth as a result of irreversible anoxia. This was tragedy enough but worse compounded by the mother having had a fruitless major operation.

A careful watch was kept immediately after delivery for post-partum haemorrhage due to reduced clotting factors. This was done with the aid of the haematological laboratory. Later the output of urine was monitored to detect the possible early onset of renal failure and anuria. If the patient could be kept alive for about ten days there was the possibility of recovery of renal function. Eric George Lapthorne Bywaters (b.1910) with others in 1941 showed in crush syndrome due to injury that controlling the intake of fluid and nutrients exactly to match the output could preserve the lives of patients until kidney function returned. There had to be most careful monitoring of fluid output, especially insensible losses of water and that lost by vomiting. Intake by gastric tube into the stomach consisted of measured quanitities of fluid and concentrated nutrients – protein, fat, carbohydrate, vitamins and minerals – to maintain metabolism at acceptable levels.

The method was used with some success in cases of anuria due to abruptio. Slightly later such patients were transferred to special units for renal dialysis, mainly by appropriate machines made for the purpose. For a short time peritoneal dialysis was used but was superseded.

It came to be believed that abruptio might in some way be due to deficiency of folic acid. This was one of the reasons for the routine administration of this vitamin during pregnancy. The other reason was, of course, the prevention of macrocytic anemia.

Pre-eclampsia and eclampsia

The patho-physiology of these conditions remained a mystery, despite myriad attempts in blood and biochemical analysis, and measurements of blood flows in a variety of organs, and several more esoteric investigations. Enormously long books detailed all of these and there were hundreds of learned articles, but the causes of pre-eclampsia and eclampsia resisted elucidation despite all efforts. It was appropriately called the 'disease of theories'. The approach to dealing with it therefore had to be empirically clinical rather than based on demonstrable agreed scientific fact.

There are no subjective symptoms of pre-eclampsia. The physical signs are those of raised blood pressure, proteinuria and oedema. These were sought deliberately at every antenatal visit. Special areas in printed clinical notes were reserved for them to be recorded. Weight gain too, as a possible sign of increased water retention, was recorded. More than 0.5kg per week for the last 28 weeks of pregnancy was taken to mean evidence of excessive water retention, though whether this might or might not be significant was not entirely estalished. It came to be accepted that any rise of blood pressure above 140 mmHg systolic and 90 mmHg diastolic were usually the first indicators of the disorder, requiring immediate admission to hospital. There had been too many cases where this advice was ignored in which the blood pressure rose to near-fatal or fatal heights in a matter of hours. There was no way in which this could then be forecast.

Proteinuria too is a potentially serious matter. It might be the first sign of trouble to come, foreshadowing a rapid rise in blood pressure. Oedema alone, over the tibiae, was less serious clinically but if of rapid onset might be the earliest sign presaging raised blood pressure and/or proteinuria. With such uncertainty in forecasting the progress of the disease the only thing to do was to play safe. That invariably meant admission to hospital for rest and observation.

Rest in bed, perhaps supplemented with some sedative, was often the best and most effective treatment in early cases. Physical activity allied with anxiety may be causes of increased blood pressure. With these two minimized the blood pressure may fall, often quite significantly. Moreover rest in bed tends to increase urine flow and so perhaps diminish water retention, though the role of this in the genesis of pre-eclampsia was problematical.

Monitoring of the blood pressure at least twice a day and often more frequently, testing of the urine for protein at least once a day, and search for oedema as well as daily weighing were part of the hospital regime. Ophthalmoscopic examination was often helpful for there may be changes in the retina and retinal vessels. The onset of serious disease and of eclampsia does have vague subjective symptoms of headache, flashes of light and difficulty in reading, and a feeling of being unwell. Jaundice may show the onset of liver failure, and falling urine output may presage renal failure. All these signs and symptoms were looked for and gave indications of remorseless progress of the disease, or more happily whether it was being held in check or better still regressing.

With regression to normal there were a few women who could be safely allowed to go home and attend antenatal clinics frequently. In those in whom the pre-eclampsia seemed stationary the conservative hospital regime had to be continued. Attempts were often made to use diuretics such as chlorothiazide, and hypotensive drugs but these last did not seem to be very effective. Moreover there was always the fear that although the maternal blood pressure might be reduced by them there was no certainty that they improved the maternal placental blood flow. It is on this that the life and health of the fetus depend. Some patients on hypotensives seemed to lose their babies despite apparently having their blood pressures controlled.

What to do if the disease worsened depended on the rate of progression. If the pregnancy had continued to within a week or two of term and the baby seemed clinically mature and the clinical signs were not advancing too rapidly then the usual course was to induce labour by rupturing the membranes. During labour sedation had to be intensified as compared with normal, as also did analgesia so that fits should be prevented. There was anxiety about using a Syntocinon drip, but this misgiving was probably unnecessary. It dated from earlier times when Pitressin contained both oxytocin and vasopressin. This last undoubtedly raises blood pressure. But Syntocinon (oxytocin) is free of it, and alone does not cause an increase in blood pressure.

Labour, in these cases, was carefully monitored, especially as regards the blood pressure. Anaesthesia had to be readily available in case of the potential onset of eclampsia. Fits had to be prevented at all costs. If they occurred the prognosis for life for both mother and baby worsened rapidly. It was often wisest to deliver the baby with forceps under general anaesthesia to minimize the painful stimuli which might precipitate a fit. Serious deterioration of the woman's condition was shown by rapidly rising blood pressure, sometimes to above 120 mm Hg diastolic. The urine might be solid with the heavy precipitate of protein on boiling and adding a drop or two of acetic acid. Oedema could become widespread causing bloating of the face and gross swelling of the hands, feet and legs. This set of signs came to be recognized as 'imminent eclampsia'. Rapid action was necessary, and was obviously seen to be so. Both lives were at serious risk. In this emergency general anaesthesia was induced either before or as soon as the patient could be taken to the operating theatre, where caesarean section was undertaken, whatever the length of the pregnancy. Sometimes this might be as early as 29 weeks with a baby weighing 1kg or less. Yet it still had a better chance of survival in the Special Care Nursery than staying in the womb. It was well expressed that in such severe cases the woman was harbouring a dangerous endocrine tumour which had to be removed, just as any similar dangerous tumour would be. The fact that the tumour was a baby with its placenta was beside the point, especially as caesarean section was the best treatment for both patients.

All patients with pre-eclampsia/eclampsia needed the same careful monitoring after delivery as before it. The serious cases were not out of danger of developing eclampsia till about a week had passed. Hypotensive drugs could be used with greater impunity in the puerperium since there was now no worry about any effects on the baby. Sedation could be maintained almost continuously too, as required by the clinical condition. Despite the empiricism of this monitoring and treatment for all degrees of pre-eclampsia/eclampsia the results for both mother and baby improved enormously during this period. It is not uncommon to be able to deal effectively with problems, both medical and otherwise, without full scientific understanding of their nature. Some things require action before their scientific bases can be fully comprehended.

Pre-eclampsia/eclampsia can develop on a background of essential hypertension and renal disease. These may be diagnosed early in pregnancy, and perhaps treated on lines that would be used if the woman were not pregnant. If this should be successful then most careful monitoring is still needed to detect the early onset of pre-eclampsia later in the pregnancy. Both hypertension and renal disease may deteriorate in pregnancy, sometimes because of it. This may be accepted by women, their husbands and attendants, as good reasons for abortion, early delivery by caesarean section or early induction of labour at any time. Physical, psychological and social factors have to be taken into account in these very difficult decisions.

There is an increased tendency to develop pre-eclampsia in subsequent pregnancies when it has occurred in previous ones. This may give pause for thought in what to do about contraception and limiting the size of the family. Even sterilization might have to be considered. Yet even in the most severe cases of pre-eclampsia/eclampsia there may be no recurrence in subsequent pregnancies. It is wise therefore to be most conservative in prognosis. It might be best to go ahead with a pregnancy and see what happens. That may in fact be nothing untoward, the pregancy and delivery being quite normal. Prognosis is in these cases statistical. There is a tendency to be too pessimistic about the risk in individuals, for in a second pregnancy the disorder may recur in 25 per cent of those who suffered it in a first pregnancy. That means that three-quarters will not develop it again. The only way to find out is to try, and treat any consequences as they arise. However in third pregnancies, with two previous ones complicated by pre-eclampsia, the risk of recurrence rises to 50 per cent and to 75 or 100 per cent in fourth and fifth pregnancies.

On the basis of the clinical findings it seemed that pre-eclampsia/eclampsia was a response of the cardiovascular system to a variety of physiological (and perhaps pathological) factors, probably in combination, due to the metabolic and other changes inseparable from pregnancy. The nature of these factors could only be matters for conjecture. Generalized vascular contraction, raising the peripheral resistance, seemed to be the cause of raised blood pressure. More localized vascular spasm in the kidneys might be the proximate cause of proteinuria. Localized spasm in the liver might be the cause of jaundice, and in the brain the cause of headache and subjective feelings of flashes of light, when eclampsia was imminent. Diminished blood flow to the placenta, because of vascular contraction, seemed to be the likely cause for the poor fetal growth so often seen with prolonged raised blood pressure. It is a definite association with the small-for-dates babies.

Oedema could only be due to excessive fluid in the extra-vascular space, not necessarily due to excessive total water retention. Fluid might exude from the blood or the cells of many organs and tissues. This last demanded as an explanation some change in the permeability of cell membranes, moving water out of cells and into the surrounding extracellular fluid. But the underlying causes of all these clinical phenomena had to await further investigation and understanding as they still do now. Until the cause or causes can be determined and treated, management must remain on empirical lines which have been shown over several decades to be largely successful clinically.

Eclampsia became rare because of the tight hospital control of the underlying disorder. When it did occur it was treated on the lines originating with Stroganoff. However, chloroform was never used as an anaesthetic since it is a liver poison and might precipitate failure of that organ, already damaged by the disease, causing severe jaundice and almost certain death. There was readier recourse to the use of caesarean section if only one or two fits had occurred in pregnancy or early labour. This offered the best prognosis for both mother and child. With the baby delivered sedation could be massively intensified to protect the mother from further fits. She could be kept almost continuously narcotised for several days as a prophylaxis against recurrent fits and their serious danger to her life.

For a long time it was erroneously believed that pre-eclampsia/eclampsia could have permanent after-effects by causing chronic renal disease or continuing hypertension. This has been shown to be untrue and the whole symptom and sign complex now seems to be confined entirely to pregnancy and the puerperium with no mater consequences. But serious anuria or liver failure may be exceptions to this.

Obstetric operations and interventions

External version

This conversion of a breech presentation or a transverse lie to a cephalic presentation, by abdominal manipulation, was used whenever it seemed likely to be successful. There had to be some mobility of the fetus within the uterus and its contained liquor amnii. This was more likely in transverse lie, the mother often being multiparous, so that she had a lax uterus and much liquor. The problem, however, is not that of turning the baby but making it stay put as a cephalic presentation. That demands uterine contractions forcing the head into the pelvis. Often this could only be brought about by labour. With a very unstable lie, constantly recurring after version, the only recourse was to admit the mother to hospital, turn the baby, rupture the membranes and put up a Syntocinon drip to get her to go into labour.

In breech presentations, especially when the legs were extended, version might be impossible. The cone shaped bottom is pushed down into the pelvic brim, by a taut uterus, and cannot be pulled up into the abdomen. Such a presentation is most likely in a primigravida having a fairly tense uterus in the last few weeks of pregnancy, There is no point in persisting if this is the case. The manipulation may be worth a try, but excessive force is unwarranted and dangerous. Even in the easy cases the placenta may be partially separated from the uterine wall, or the umbilical cord, especially if long, may be entangled round the baby's body, limbs or neck and seriously diminish the fetal blood supply.

If the baby in either of these conditions cannot be turned and made stable in the new presentation, consideration has to be given to the safest way to effect delivery. Caesarean section is often the best choice. A transverse lie in labour can be a dire disaster and must be avoided for the safety of both mother and baby. Breech vaginal delivery, on the other hand, can often be safely undertaken. However, there is no doubt that the fetal mortality from breech delivery is higher than that from cephalic delivery, particularly if the pelvis is not large. It requires more obstetric skill than delivery with the head coming first. There are fewer and fewer obstetricians with the necessary competence for vaginal breech delivery, now that more and more caesarean sections are being performed. This freer use of abdominal section has virtually done away with many of the old obstetric skills. On balance, however, it is probably a gain. Internal version, destructive operations and *accouchement forcée* were used when matters in labour had progressed so far as to endanger the mother's life. With the increasing safety of caesarean section none of them were acceptable to the professionals or the people they served. Otiose skills were best left to wither.

Amniocentesis

Withdrawal of amniotic fluid using a long needle passed through the abdominal wall into the uterus was increasingly used. At first it was done 'blind', that is without knowing where the placenta was situated. In some cases it was inevitably pierced. Sometimes abortion was caused, and sometimes haemorrhage. But a serious effect was when fetal blood leaked into the maternal circulation. This was a sure way to cause the formation of maternal antibodies if the mother were Rhesus negative and her baby Rhesus positive. The baby might then develop Rhesus disease. Locating the placenta was therefore increasingly done by the use of ultrasound. The needle could then be passed by a route to avoid it.

Liquor was investigated for its cellular, enzyme and other biochemical content. Cells shed by the fetus into the liquor can be sexed by the chromatin of their nuclei. Some disorders are sex-linked so that it was possible to identify fetuses liable to be affected. In some cases the affected fetuses were aborted if the parents wished it after they knew of the risks. Alpha-fetoprotein levels in the liquor helped to confirm the likelihood of central nervous system maldevelopment. Bile pigments were used to assess the severity of erythroblastosis fetalis. Enzyme content helped diagnose some rare inherited disorders. Hyaline membrane disease or respiratory distress syndrome in the newborn was estimated to be likely or not by determining the lecithin-sphingomyelin ratio in the liquor near term or in early labour. The disorder could sometimes be prevented by administering a corticosteroid to the mother.

This is by no means an exhaustive list of the investigations made on specially withdrawn liquor. It can be seen from these trends that its examination came to give more and more information about the fetus. Every passing month seemed to bring another test devised for intrauterine diagnosis, and still the investigations multiply. They demand the cooperation of neonatal paediatricians, geneticists, biochemists and pathologists. It is unfortunate that not always could specific treatment follow diagnosis, but at least forewarned was to be forearmed to do what was physically possible for the baby and also to be prepared to counsel parents so that their suffering might be minimized.

Intra-uterine fetal diagnosis thus progressed apace. Its justification lies in the probability that effective treatments, either before or after birth, will be devised as knowledge increases. It is the usual form of progress in understanding diseases that first they are characterized and only later become capable of treatment. The whole history of medicine attests to this generalization.

Chorionic villus sampling

A more direct method of genetic sexing of cells, and therefore the embryo and fetus, was chorionic villus sampling. Early in pregnancy the chorion, from which the placenta later develops, is easily accessible through the cervix. Small pieces of chorion can be withdrawn and sexing accurately is more sure than it can be on cells shed into the amniotic cavity. Later in pregnancy the site of the placenta can be shown by ultrasound. A needle thrust into its substance can withdraw a few cells, sufficient for investigation.

Intra-uterine transfusion

A special application of amniocentesis was the injection of blood into the peritoneal cavity of the fetus when it was seriously affected by Rhesus disease. This, by haemolysis, causes progressive and ultimately fatal anaemia in the baby. It was discovered that some red cells injected into the peritoneum could be absorbed into the blood stream and to some extent alleviate the anaemia. When this was the case the fetus might be allowed to remain in utero for a little longer before delivery. Such prolongation gave a chance for the fetus to become more mature and therefore more likely to survive after birth.

Fetoscopy

Of course peritoneal transfusion cannot be as effective as direct transfusion into a vein of the fetus. Attempts were made to do this in otherwise hopeless cases. Under direct vision, using a lighted special telescope similar to a cystoscope, a vein can be found on the surface of the placenta, and with great difficulty a needle can be inserted into it through which a transfusion of blood may be given. It is likely that over the years the technique will become increasingly possible and more successful. Another use for the fetoscope was found in directly visualising the fetus to look for abnormalities of the limbs, abdominal wall and nervous system.

Fetal surgery

A further advance has been the recent attempts to correct some surgical conditions by operating on the fetus in utero. It is not yet widely practised but as with other surgical advances the techniques will be improved, standardized and come to be accepted as normal and proper interventions.

There are great problems to be solved in this form of surgery. One of the main ones is that the amniotic cavity has to be opened. That allows for escape of the liquor and the uterus contracts down to attempt to expel all the uterine contents through the incision, so that it may not be possible to get the fetus back inside the uterus after the procedure. However, these problems are slowly being overcome. Just as undreamt of interventions were made in thoracic, cardiac and neurological surgery in the recent past and have now become acceptable and routine, so will intrauterine surgery progress along similar lines. Apart from the technical problems there will be economic, moral and ethical ones to be solved. It is these which will probably determine the rate of progress in this most recent surgical and obstetric advance into the unknown.

Induction of labour

Efficacious medical inductions were sought. If they work they are obviously better than breaching the membranes which allows bacteria into the interior of the uterus and to the baby. Prostaglandin pessaries in the vagina seemed often to be of value for this purpose. Oxytocin intravenous drips sometimes served. The older methods of castor oil and quinine were abandoned, though an enema alone often brought the woman to start in labour and had the advantage of emptying the bowel. Pharmacological advances will in the future find safe simple and certain methods of inducing labour.

If the indications made it certain that the woman must be started in labour, then, under sedation, the cervix was stretched with fingers, the forewaters ruptured, and an oxytocin drip set up. This is surgical induction. If this failed to work after about 48 hours then intra-uterine infection was almost inevitable. Bacteriological swabs were therefore taken at 24 hours and at intervals thereafter, in case antibiotics and chemotherapy were needed, to prevent puerperal sepsis and infection in the baby.

Failed induction sometimes meant that a caesarean section had to be performed. The indications for undertaking the induction therefore had to be sound and not just for the convenience of the patient or professional attendants. The commonest indication was perhaps postmaturity. After 42 weeks of pregnancy there is a rising curve of fetal and neonatal mortality, probably due to relative failure of placental functions. Babies can become very large too if they stay in the uterus long past the normal time. This can be a cause of difficulty and obstruction in labour. Before the use of ultrasound it was easy to make clinical mistakes in deciding when pregnancy was prolonged. The exact timing of the length of pregnancy and measurements of the size of the fetal head by ultrasound made the diagnosis of postmaturity very sure, when before it had been based on clinical grounds of dubious accuracy.

Caesarean section

The technique of caesarean section was established. It was virtually always done through the lower segment of the uterus. This keeps the scar in the uterus out of the peritoneal cavity, since the peritoneal flap on the upper part of the bladder is sewn over it. If infection should occur it is less serious in this situation than if it is within the peritoneal cavity. The site of the incision in the uterus also heals well because it is in a relatively quiescent part during the puerperium. Experience showed that in a subsequent pregnancy and labour rupture of the uterus occurred four times more commonly in classical section scars, made in the body of the uterus, than when the former incision was in the lower segment. The classical upper segment caesarean section was therefore abandoned.

The longitudinal incision in the adbominal wall, running from the umbilicus down to the pubis was also abandoned in favour of the transverse one described originally by Pfannenstiel, running just above the pubic hair line. Women much preferred this more cosmetic incision which could easily be kept out of sight by clothing, especially beachwear.

The indications for caesarean section widened enormously. It became commonplace for hospitals to deliver ten per cent of women by the operation. In some American practices the rate rose to 25 per cent. The reasons were various, but the main one was perhaps to be sure of delivering a live baby. The risks were thought to be great for the baby in conditions such as antepartum haemorrhage; pre-eclampsia; breech and other malpresentations and malpositions; postmaturity; minor degrees of disproportion; many intercurrent diseases, especially diabetes; small-for-dates babies and many other problems, including fetal distress in the first stage of labour. The operation carried very little risk for mothers, so was increasingly done for the sake of the baby.

In past centuries, and even earlier in the 20th century, the risks of caesarean section for the mother were deemed to be too great to be countenanced purely for the sake of the baby. Only about after 1950 did the balance swing greatly in favour of the fetus, because the mother could be safely cared for during and after caesarean section.

Reinforcing the readier recourse to caesarean section was the widespread belief among the public and the professionals, that every pregnancy should result in a healthy mother and a healthy baby. Everything had to be done to make sure that this happened.

It was an expectation of perfection, which could never be guaranteed, though people behaved as if it could be. The result was that obstetricians doubted their purely obstetric skills in dealing with the problems of labour in the old ways. They knew their limitations there, because of lack of practice, but they were confident about their competence in caesarean section. When this was performed it was thought by all that everything possible had been done and that no one was to blame for anything that might go wrong. And this belief in the achievability of perfection resulted in increased litigation against obstetricians when things did go wrong and the baby might die, or be damaged for life. All these factors operated in causing the increase in caesarean sections. It was often thought to be negligent if the obstetrician did not perform a caesarean section if the outcome of a vaginal delivery was a dead or damaged baby. Proving legal negligence became a happy hunting ground for aggrieved unhappy saddened parents and their lawyers. It was understandable but sapped the confidence of obstetricians in their own abilities and competence. Perfection is not attainable, yet that is what they and their patients strove for and expected. Increased numbers of caesarean sections were the result of these laudable yet finally unachievable aims.

Of course there were many who deplored this increase in operative delivery, not least obstetricians and midwives. But there were particularly active and vociferous women's groups who insisted that the trend had gone too far. They were certainly right in some instances, for sometimes the operation was done on the flimsy grounds of convenience for the mother or her family, or even to avoid inconvenience for the obstetrician, perhaps having to get up at night to go to his patient. Almost the slightest deviation from what was taken to be normal, perhaps erroneously, came to excuse the use of abdominal delivery. It was said, with some truth, that male obstetricians were taking over women's bodies and imposing 'medicalization' of childbirth. Many midwives agreed. This led to many women opting for home delivery in the heart of the family and with only a midwife, perhaps supported by a general practitioner, in attendance. When all goes well this is truly ideal, but because of the unpredictability and swift deterioration of many complications both during pregnancy and childbirth, it can on occasion be very hazardous both for mother and baby. The arguments continue to rage, but are not resolved. There is so much to be said with truth on either side of these conflicting policies. Some emphasize one set of circumstances and some another to support their arguments and beliefs.

What has emerged, however, is that the place of delivery and the sort of care she receives should be determined by the woman herself, though in proper consultation with her intended assistants. The problem here is that all of them may err, mislead and be misled. That is inseparable from all medical practice, but errors of physical care are very much less likely in the hospital environment, which is better suited to dealing with clinical problems and emergencies as they arise. On the other hand hospital care is often sadly lacking in full communication and psychological understanding of the reproducing woman.

There is obvious need for fuller cooperation between domiciliary and hospital services so that every woman shall feel she receives the best physical and the best psychological care available in her vicinity. This is a question of management which should arrange facilities to the best advantage for each woman, heeding what she wants. But it has to be said that many women prefer the physical safety of hospital care as against the psychological benefits of home delivery. With appropriate advice they should be allowed to choose what they believe will suit them best without undue pressure being brought to bear on them. But it has to be remembered that the price of a healthy baby and a healthy mother, in the physical sense, is unremitting close attention throughout pregnancy and labour and after, by conscientious and well-trained competent professionals. Neither a dead mother nor a dead baby has any psychology. Excellent physical care is therefore paramount, though that need not mean that the psychological welfare of the woman is neglected, as it has undoubtedly been in the recent past.

Obstetric radiology

There was a sharp decline in the use of radiology in pregnancy and labour, because of its dangers to the fetus. X-rays were found to be a cause of malformations in the baby if the embryo was exposed to them. Moreover there was good evidence that relatively excesive exposure of the fetus to X-rays in pregnancy, such as those for routine pelvimetry, was a cause of leukaemia developing in childhood. The indications for radiography therefore had to be very sure, in the belief that information could be gained in no other way. In many instances sonar or ultrasound had provided that other way.

Radiology was still used for the diagnosis of fetal malformations such as spina bifida, hydrocephaly, anencephaly and limb defects. It could provide almost certain evidence of multiple pregnancy too. None of these usually needed more than a single exposure to X-rays so any danger was kept to a minimum.

A single radiograph too was all that was needed to confirm or deny the presence of disproportion at term. The clinical diagnosis of this can often be uncertain when it appears that the head will not engage fully in the pelvic brim, nor be made to do so by downward pressure from the abdomen. A lateral radiograph can show the exact measurement of the size of the pelvic brim antero-posteriorly, and the widest diameter of the head can also often be measured. These two together can be a valuable indication of disproportion. The film may also show that either the brow or face are presenting. All these may modify decisions about how the baby shall be delivered.

A rare use of X-rays is in cases of hydramnios to show the presence of oesophageal atresia in the fetus. Normally some liquor is disposed of by fetal swallowing. This cannot occur in oesophageal atresia so that fluid accumulates. The injection of a radio-opaque dye into the liquor can show that the fetal oesophagus is blocked or narrowed for even such a malformed fetus swallows some of the fluid and its contained dye.

The place of radiography was largely taken over by ultrasound. After some initial anxieties this technique was shown to be without harm to the fetus so that it could be employed with impunity. It can be used for the early diagnosis of pregnancy by seeing the embryo and recording the heart beat. It can give a diagnosis of embryonic death and whether the uterus is empty after an abortion. It is most valuable in measuring the bi-parietal diameter of the head at all stages of pregnancy and so estimate normal or abormal growth of the fetus. Location of the placenta, the position of the head, the diagnosis of multiple pregnancy and many malformations are well within its compass. It has turned out to be one of the major advances in obstetrics for decades, even centuries. Due honour should be accorded to Professor Ian Donald, of Glasgow, for its introduction. Almost single-handedly it was he who started the technique and in the early days developed it. As a result of this work in obstetrics it has been imported as a diagnostic tool into almost every other branch of medicine. Its applications increase almost by the month.

Labour

First stage

The outstanding feature in the management of the first stage of labour at this time was the increased monitoring of progress. Maternal factors to be taken into account were her mental state, pulse, blood pressure and fluid balance, as well as regular testing of the urine for protein. These gave indications of whether she was becoming distressed. Uterine contractions were assessed for their strength, frequency and duration. These gave indications of whether they were progressing normally, or whether they were relatively inert or stormy. Either of these two last suggested the possibility of some degree of obstruction to the passage of the fetus through the bony pelvis. The assessment of the contractions could usually be made clinically, even though it might appear somewhat imprecise. Strength was estimated on hardness at the height of contractions. Frequency was easy enough to measure as being the number of contractions in a given time, usually ten or 15 minutes. The onset and cessation of contractions are difficult to define, though the woman herself knows their onset. Cessation is more indefinite. Nevertheless one observer can successfully monitor changes of the contractions making it of value in deciding if they are normal, falling away or getting stronger.

In some advanced units the characteristics of uterine contractions were recorded graphically. A simple strain gauge tokodynamometer was strapped to the abdomen. It provided a written record of the contractions, their strength, frequency and duration. Progress in descent of the head was estimated to some degree by abdominal palpation. The upper part of the head where it meets the neck can usually be defined. Its height above the pubis can be recorded. The amount of the head within the pelvis was estimated in fifths, so that three-fifths meant that the head was engaged, with two-fifths remaining above the symphysis.

The lie, presentation and position were known from abdominal palpation at the start of labour. The fetal heart rate was regularly recorded every 15 minutes or so using abdominal auscultation clinically. The normal range was from 120 to 160 beats per minute in between contractions. During contractions the fetal heart slowed, though it was difficult to estimate the time taken for the return to normal after the contraction. This became more precise with the introduction of fetal electrocardiography.

Prior to this time it had been difficult to disentangle the electrical activity of the heart of the fetus from that of its mother. Clever computerization of the combined records allowed that of the mother to be cancelled out if recordings were taken from the abdomen. Then the fetal heart rate could easily be calculated and recorded from second to second. Graphically the rate was recorded continuously. During contractions the rate fell, normally wth quick recovery. These were designated Type I dips. But when recovery was slow they were called Type II dips. These presaged fetal distress and could be a serious sign of fetal anoxia. Recurrent Type II dips usually meant that it was best for the fetus to be delivered almost immediately, by caesarean section if the cervix was not fully dilated, and perhaps by forceps if it was fully open. Recording from scalp electrodes applied through the partially open cervix gave direct readings of fetal heart activity, with little interference from the mother's electrocardiogram.

Regular digital vaginal examinations, probably about every four to six hours, were an essential part of the monitoring. These determined the taking up of the cervix, its thinning and the rate of dilatation. The firm application of the head to the cervix all around its circumference was a good sign of a well flexed head. Whether the membranes were ruptured was important and noted. The descent of the head, if not distorted by *caput succedaneum* (oedema and swelling of the scalp) or moulding of the skull bones as they were compressed, gave evidence of descent. If the vertex descended to the level of the ischial spines, which could easily be felt, then the major part of the head had passed through the pelvic brim, and was therefore engaged.

The boggy swelling of the *caput succedaneum* on the head was a sign that the head was undergoing some degree of compression, perhaps due to mild disproportion. The overriding of the skull bones, moulding, meant that the head was being severely compressed by disproportion. This should have been recognized earlier and prevented perhaps by caesarean section. Palpation of the sutures and fontanelles determined the site of the occiput in relation to the pelvis, and whether the head was deflexed, as in an occipito-posterior or brow presentation. And of course face presentations could be determined by vaginal palpation.

In cases of doubt about fetal anoxia it became possible to take small samples of blood from the accessible scalp when the cervix was open. These were tested for their pH to give an indication of serious shortage of circulating oxygen. The fetal electrocardiogram could also be recorded by electrodes fastened to the scalp. As a result of these investigations the diagnosis of fetal distress was made certain, rather than as a result of clinical impression based entirely on interpretation of the fetal heart rate.

The close monitoring made it possible to diagnose maternal distress, fetal distress or delay in progress. Often all three combined. Maternal distress alone might be alleviated with drugs or even an epidural anaesthetic if the main cause of her symptoms was pain. But more than this might call for caesarean section. Fetal distress called for caesarean section too, immediate if the cord prolapsed. There is no knowing just how long a fetus may withstand anoxia without death or later impairment. On those grounds almost immediate caesarean section is justified.

Failure to progress is rather harder to judge. If the head fails to descend into the pelvis and/or the cervix fails to dilate further over the course of a few hours, especially if accompanied by caput succedaneum or moulding, then caesarean section was done. The timing of decision was also influenced by the strength of the uterine contractions and the physiological responses of the mother and fetus. If it were certain that any delay was not due to serious disproportion then an oxytocin drip was tried. This might stimulate the uterine contractions and a successful delivery eventuate.

It used to be an invariable rule that if the cervix was not fully dilated then the only safe means of delivery was by caesarean section. But about this time there was developed, by Malmstrom of Sweden, an effective suction-tractor, or ventouse. It was not the first of its kind for James Young Simpson had tried to devise one. In the new ventouse a metal cup was applied to the scalp through the cervix. A pump slowly evacuating the air from the cup drew the scalp into it so that a complete seal was formed. A chain attached to the cup could then be used to exert traction on the head through the pull on the scalp. It was sometimes used just before the cervix was fully dilated and seemed capable of helping to dilate it and then draw the head down through the vagina to be delivered.

There were many enthusiasts for the ventouse. It was said to be completely safe even in the hands of those who were not competent with the obstetric forceps, that is some general practitioners and midwives. On the other hand were those who had seen damage to the brain as a result of head compression and distortion. The great pull on the scalp can in turn be transmitted to the skull and its contents. The instrument came to have a small place in dealing with problems just before full dilatation of the cervix, but after full dilatation there is little doubt that forceps were more efficacious and safer, in competent hands. Before full dilatation the answer was virtually always caesarean section.

The sometimes excessive monitoring of progress, especially when recording instruments or an oxytocin drip were used, again turned many women away from hospital delivery. They saw every intervention, often rightly, as an interference with the proper course of labour. They resented the constant interference, often by male doctors. They wanted simply to be left alone with a midwife and be allowed to get on with it in their own way. But a balance has to be struck. Mothers and fetuses do get distressed and labour does sometimes fail to progress, however determined the mother, and however well prepared. Intervention is then undoubtedly necessary in a modern culture. That intervention has to be based in sound principles and exact observations. These are the justification for the monitoring even with electronic recording instruments.

If a caesarean, ventouse or forceps delivery has to be done then the indications should be as definite as they can be made. There should be a proper reluctance to proceed to any form of operative delivery, or an oxytocin drip, until it is sure that nothing else will serve. Getting the balance right is by no means easy. Some patients and their assistants wait too long before intervening and some intervene too easily. Either may have serious consequences. Finding the right moment has to be based in clinical and patient judgment supported by as many facts as possible. It is the search for those facts and their interpretation that so disturbs many women. Also the facts derived from electronic monitoring are not as incontrovertible as might at first seem. They do need sceptical understanding before being accepted as right. They too can be wrong and/ or wrongly interpreted.

The other cause for women's concern was the too free use of sedation, analgesics and anaesthetics. It was usual to give sedatives during the early part of the first stage, and then as the pain increased to use pethidine intramuscular injections, repeated as seemed necessary. Gas and air or gas and oxygen, or trilene, might be administered in the most painful phase just before full dilatation. In cases of extreme pain an anaesthetist might be called in to give an epidural anaesthetic.

Those who had undergone 'natural childbirth' training resented these interferences which, to them, often seemed to be dictated by professionals. But even those who have trained themselves sometimes suffer very great pain, and many of them properly cry for help to ease it. There is no doubt that no sedative, analgesic or anaesthetic should be given without full consultation with the patient. She should know about them and be taught about them and their purposes before labour ever begins. Then she can participate in the decisions about when to use them so that she may 'consult her own ease'. Labour pains are not a punishment to be borne under all circumstances, when they can be alleviated by modern technological advances. Sedatives and analgesics are used in vast quantities for a variety of medical and surgical conditions. There is no need to make an emotional irrational exception of labour.

Second stage

This became a more or less standard procedure from the point of view of the attendants. The woman was on her back, though in a few units on her left side. It had to be made sure that the cervix was truly fully dilated by vaginal examination. Allowing the woman to push on an undilated cervix, even a small anterior lip, had been known for centuries to be a potent cause of trouble, the cervix becoming massively oedematous and obstructing labour.

At full dilatation there was then encouragement to push with every contraction. Too often this was vociferous and out of keeping with the occasion. Light-hearted irrelevant conversation between attendants, sometimes excluding the patient, was frequently heard. It was thoughtless, seeming to upstage the woman who should have felt herself to be the centre of attention. At the height of contractions gas and air or gas and oxygen, or trilene were administered by the patient herself if she wished it.

After every contraction the fetal heart was listened to and counted. In the general excitement and concern for the mother it was all too easy to forget the incipient dangers of fetal anoxia. Slow recovery of the heart rate to normal was an indication for forceps, or more rarely ventouse, delivery. One of the worst tragedies of obstetrics is when the fetus dies in the few minutes before birth.

It was unusual to allow the second stage to last more than about one hour. In the early part of this period it was taken to be normal for this stage to last up to two hours. That was really too long. The progress of descent of the head was usually obvious enough for the scalp could be seen at the vulva. Sometimes vaginal examination was needed for this assessment.

As the perineum stretched in front of the distending head it might be seen to begin to split at the fourchette. This was an indication to perform a small episiotomy, the cut being from the fourchette to the outer part of the dark area surrounding the anus. This was enough to prevent a tear extending into the anal sphincter, or beyond that into the anus and rectum.

The timing of the episiotomy and its extent were often misjudged. If done too early it was ineffective in aiding delivery of the head, which was its main purpose, and it allowed undue bleeding to occur. If left too late then a severe tear might result. Many episiotomies were made too big and several too small. The nice judgement required depended on training and clinical experience. But not infrequently it was done injudiciously. Moreover it was done too often, and quite rightly that caused public disquiet in women's organizations. Patience on the part of the attendants often allowed progressive stretching of the perineum so that damage to it did not occur as the head delivered.

The perineum was 'supported' by a hand over a pad covering the anus. It was supposed to prevent tearing, though that is doubtful. It was also thought to aid full flexion of the head so that its smallest possible diameter came through the vulval orifice. This too was of doubtful efficacy. But there was some merit in preventing soiling of the area from the anus, and in helping to bring about, as far as possible a gentle slow delivery of the head.

As the head 'crowned', that is as its widest diameter distended the vulva, an injection of intramuscular syntometrine was given. This contained oxytocin and ergometrine, both designed to cause contractions of the uterus, aiding it to separate and expel the placenta. It was a most valuable practice.

After the head emerged the eyes were wiped gently and the mouth cleared of mucus, by a suction catheter if need be. A few more contractions and pushes rotated the shoulders so that they were antero-posterior at the outlet. Gentle backward traction on the head brought the anterior shoulder into view and moving the head forwards allowed delivery of the posterior shoulder, and thereafter the body and legs of the fetus slid out of the birth canal.

The baby was held up by the feet, supposedly to allow liquor to drain out of its upper air passages. The mouth was sucked out with a catheter. The umbilical cord was clamped or tied twice about 3" from the navel, and then cut through. The baby was wrapped in a sheet and should always have been handed to the mother if all was well. But even here thoughtlessness crept in and the baby was often whisked away to a cot and just as rapidly removed to the nursery to be weighed. It was as if the baby belonged to the midwives and not the mother. Gradually and fortunately this practice changed, giving the mother her baby as soon as it was born. But it is astonishing that the thoughtless practice was not realized earlier and that it took patient groups to draw attention to it.

Forceps delivery

The indications for forceps delivery were maternal distress, fetal distress or delay in delivery. A common form of delay was due to 'deep tranverse arrest' where the occiput stayed in the transverse position and could not be forced to rotate to the anterior position by the muscular efforts of the mother. To deal with this it was usual in the early part of this period to administer a general anaesthetic. In favourable cases the 'half hand' of four fingers in the vagina could rotate the head anteriorly and then forceps could be applied to effect delivery. Later it was more common to use Kielland's forceps which were ideal for application directly to the right place on the fetal head and the rotation could be brought about using them. Sometimes Kielland's were used only for rotation, followed by application of the more classical forceps for extraction. Whatever method was used a wide episotomy was always needed for the forceps otherwise distended and tore the perineum, perhaps into the anus and rectum.

Later in the period it was increasingly common to use internal pudendal nerve block as the local anaesthesia rather than general anaesthesia. It could be combined with infiltration of the perineal muscles and skin with local anaesthetic. This avoided the problem of general anaesthesia in causing vomiting during induction. If the vomit was inhaled it could lead to Mendelssohn's syndrome of sudden death or later chemical pneumonia. If epidural anaesthesia had been induced for severe pain late in the first stage, expulsive powers were often reduced and forceps delivery was then commonplace, and easily performed without further anaesthesia.

Forceps were also used in occipito-posterior positions where the occiput remained in the hollow of the sacrum. In many cases the forceps could be applied directly and the extraction made as an occipito-posterior. This was likely to cause some damage to the fetal head, perhaps with intracranial haemorrhage. It was often better to apply Kielland's forceps 'upside down' and then rotate the head through a semi-circle to bring the occiput anterior before delivery.

Breech delivery was as previously described, usually with forceps applied to the after-coming head, when the arms had been delivered. though the alternative was jaw-flexion-shoulder-traction. A prolapsed cord required immediate breech extraction. With the head low down in cephalic presentations Wrigley's forceps were ideal. They were easy to apply on to the head under simple local anaesthesia, and the short handles made it impossible to apply too much pressure to the head or to use excessive force in traction. Although domiciliary delivery had greatly declined in favour of hospital these were the only forceps which could reasonably be employed in the home.

Internal version, except occasionally for the second twin when external version failed, was entirely abandoned. A neglected transverse lie, even in the second stage, was delivered by caesarean section. The same applied to brow presentations with the head high above the brim despite the cervix being fully dilated and the woman being technically in the second stage of labour.

Comparatively few obstetricians used the ventouse in the second stage, though in inexperienced hands it might have been safer than a badly performed forceps delivery. However in all properly equipped and staffed hospitals there should always be someone competent enough to perform forceps deliveries in all circumstances when required.

Third stage

With Syntometrine given intramuscularly about the time of crowning it was almost invariable for the uterus to contract vigorously, separate the placenta from its walls and even force it down into the lower segment, just above the cervix. That this had happened was shown by abdominal palpation. The uterus was mobile from side to side and its upper part was above the navel. The placenta was drawn forth from the vagina by gentle traction on the cord while pushing the uterus upwards into the abdomen by a hand just above the symphysis pubis. It was called controlled cord traction. The alternative, slowly superseded, was to use the contracted uterus as a sort of plunger to push the placenta out of the birth canal. In the majority of cases only a few ounces of blood followed the placenta at delivery.

There was argument as to whether the maternal end of the cord should be clamped. Some thought that this would maintain the placenta's volume by retaining blood within it. They said that draining the blood out of the placenta through the cut end of the cord reduced its bulk, and minimized the power of the uterus to expel it. The argument was probably specious and for this purpose unimportant. However, clamping did prevent the whole area being covered in more blood than was necessary.

If the placenta were retained inside the cavity of the uterus it remained bulky and relatively immobile on abdominal examination. If there was no bleeding it was best to wait in the expectation of separation and descent of the placenta in due time. This might be aided by a further dose of Syntometrine. Gentle attempts at traction on the cord were also tried from time to time.

After about an hour it was probably best to deliver the placenta. Although no physical harm may come to most patients from waiting longer, even up to a day or two in past times, some of them gradually begin to suffer from surgical shock. Moreover the longer the placenta stays in the uterus the more likely does it become a nidus of infection. The woman too wants the whole process over. In the earlier period Credé's expression of the placenta was sometimes used, squeezing the uterus hard by two hands on the abdomen. This was found to be a cause of surgical shock and fell out of practice. If all else failed then manual removal had to be performed. It was never lightly undertaken since it can cause shock and introduce infection. Nevertheless it had to be done if there was continued bleeding or if the placenta was retained too long. It can be a difficult and dangerous operation, needing an experienced obstetrician to undertake it. Careless procedures can rupture the cervix or the uterine body.

In cases of loss of blood of more than a pint (500ml) transfusion was required with whole blood. Continued bleeding might need more Syntometrine to control it or ergometrine alone, perhaps administered intravenously for rapid action. Sometimes it was necessary to use bimanual compression. This was effected by putting a fist in the anterior fornix of the vagina and pressing the body of the uterus down on to it by a hand on the abdomen. The pressure had to be maintained until the bleeding ceased. If it did not then some form of clotting defect had to be considered and excluded by laboratory examination. An alternative to this form of bimanual compression was to lift the uterus upwards into the abdomen and compress it with two hands there. It was probably not quite as effective as the other method.

Whatever the method of delivery of the placenta it had always to be fully inspected. Sometimes it was obvious that a small part of it had torn away and remained within the uterus, and therefore liable to cause bleeding later. Or a small separate placenta (succenturiate lobe) might still remain within the uterus. It was usually enough simply to note these possibilities and wait to see what happened later. They were not normally an indication to proceed to search the uterus manually to find them. If bleeding occurred later a dilatation and curettage could be performed to deal with it and remove the remaining pieces of placenta.

Episiotomies and perineal tears

These were all too often cavalierly treated. It was commonplace for everyone to depart from the labour ward, after the placenta had been delivered, leaving a junior doctor to effect the repair of the perineum. Many midwives felt it to be beneath their dignity to help him or her by threading needles, handing instruments and mopping away any blood. In a few instances repairs were left till morning if the woman had delivered in the early hours. These practices were appalling, showing an unthinking callous indifference.

Local anaesthesia was used, infiltrating the whole area of the perineum. Rarely was there enough patience to wait ten minutes to allow it to take full effect. The wound was inspected to determine its extent. An ill-trained junior doctor or general practitioner might easily miss damage to the anal sphincter or even tears into the rectum. The whole business was often an unsupervised unmitigated shambles.

It was important to find the top of the tear in the vagina, to close it to prevent bleeding into the tissues behind it. A continuous fine catgut suture was used. With a finger pressing the rectum backwards the needle was passed laterally to pick up the edges of the levator ani on each side. They were drawn together by interrupted sutures of catgut. In amateur hands this was often done in a way to constrict the vagina, leading to narrowing and later dyspareunia. At this point it was taught that it should be possible to insert three fingers into the introit. The tissues are lax at this time and will tighten up later during the puerperium.

Below the levatores it was important to find any cut edges of the external sphincter ani. These showed by dimples in the skin. The ends of the muscles were sutured together, in front of the anus. Failure to do this might lead to some loss of control of defaecation and flatus. The skin was preferably repaired with a subcutaneous running suture to avoid the need for removal of stitches later. This nearly always caused much anxiety and even pain to the woman.

With this sometimes horrifyingly incompetent repair over, a finger was passed into the rectum to see if stitches had included its muscle and mucosa. This was a precaution often neglected with dire consequences of infection later. With all done a pad was placed over the vulva, the legs taken down from their unnatural position in lithotomy poles, the woman covered with warming blankets and if she were lucky she was given her baby to hold.

These were nightmare proceedings arising out of sheer thoughtlessness. There is no wonder that women's activists called for something much better than this. Fortunately some heed has been paid in the 1990s to their protestations. Childbirth in all its phases can be physically and emotionally traumatic enough without professionals making it worse, when they can make it so much better and more satisfying to the women they care for.

The repair of episiotomies and tears is so important for the future sexual life (woman that it should be given the surgical care and attention it deserves. It m classed as a minor operation in surgical terms but it can be one of the worst parts of childbirth for a woman. Badly done its later effects cause perineal pain, retention of urine, difficult bowel evacuation and dyspareunia. These have to be avoided if at all possible, and that can be achieved.

These first essays in surgery by junior doctors must be adequately taught and supervised until the repair can be competently and efficiently performed so that suffering at the time and afterwards are reduced to the absolute minimum attainable.

The relief of pain and anxiety

This subject has been touched on in several previous sections. Relief of pain and anxiety is an integral part of all aspects of midwifery. During normal pregnancy there are few indications for formal drug relief of pain. Some few complications like red degeneration of a fibroid or abruptio placentae can be extremely painful and need morphine derivatives. Chronic pain or discomfort such as that of backache may need the simple analgesics, but these, as all drugs, need care in use for fear that they may adversely affect the development of the baby.

Surgical induction of labour, usually with a Drew-Smythe catheter is virtually painless, though may be a cause of anxiety and distress. These were avoided as far as possible by kind reassurance, a sedative and perhaps an injection of pethidine prior to the procedure.

Relief of anxiety and pain in labour was increasingly the province of antenatal preparation on the lines first suggested by Grantly Dick Read. The woman and her partner were taught the rudiments of the understanding of the processes of pregnancy and labour and the puerperium. They were shown the labour wards and the meaning and uses of the apparatus there. Emphasis was laid on relaxation techniques and breathing exercises and control in the various stages of labour. There is no doubt that these all helped prepare a woman for easier childbearing through understanding and making her more aware of how to control her body and mind when under stress.

Virtually all antenatal clinics had such preparation classes. Many were run by midwives, others by physiotherapists, who founded the Obstetric Society of Physiotherapists. The Natural, later National, Childbirth Trust was instrumental in proselytizing for the methods of preparation and for the better professional care, both psychological and physical, of childbearing women. They provided training and education for expectant mothers. There was also the Association for the Improvement of the Maternity Services. These women's groups, both national and local, were immensely important in providing a unified consumer voice to which the providers had to pay serious attention. They showed up deficiencies in the services provided which the professionals had not even considered. It was in the 1950s and after that they were made to consider them, take them into account and implement the necessary changes. In the jargon of the time midwifery and obstetrics had become 'medicalized', so that many women felt alienated from those who were supposed fully to care for them. Changes in professional attitudes and understanding slowly came about as a result of these public pressures.

Those who had trained and prepared themselves for labour often were able to deliver their babies without any sedation or analgesia. A few women were also blessed with the ability to have a more or less painless labour without any special preparation. Yet the majority did feel the need for some help with pain relief. Sedation was usual in the early first stage, supplemented with injections of pethidine as seemed necessary. At the end of the first stage, the most painful period of labour, gas and air, gas and oxygen or trilene were administered by the woman herself using a variety of apparatus. This was often continued into the second stage.

Severe pain in the first stage often called for the use of epidural anaesthesia administered by an anaesthetist. It produced immense relief for some patients, otherwise greatly distressed. It had the slight disadvantage that expulsive muscular efforts in the second stage were often poor, leading to the need for a forceps delivery. However the anaesthesia was such that the instrumental delivery could be carried out without further pain relief.

Spinal anaesthesia was occasionally advocated in the literature, but was usually considered to be much too dangerous in its possible complications and side effects to gain wide acceptance. Such complications were perhaps rare but could be catastrophic in causing irreparable central nervous system damage. That seemed to most obstetricians to be an entirely unacceptable risk.

Episiotomy without anaesthesia was condemned as barbaric and no longer to be countenanced. In good time before delivery the site of the cut was infiltrated with local anaesthesia. If properly done this was often enough to allow repair of the incision later. Low forceps delivery with Wrigley's forceps was also often possible with simple infiltration of the perineum. Better still was internal pudendal nerve block. When well done this was often of value in straightforward mid-cavity forceps deliveries.

More complicated forceps deliveries often required general anaesthesia which was increasingly administered by properly trained anaesthetists. It came to be accepted by them as an operation of some magnitude needing competence and skill to avoid serious respiratory complications.

General anaesthesia was mostly used for caesarean section. It was kept light with the mother fully oxygenated to preserve the baby from the dangers of anoxia. After its delivery the anaesthesia could be deepened for the phase of repair of the uterine incision and that in the abdominal wall. A relaxant administerd with the anaesthetic made access for the surgeon to the lower uterine segment somewhat easier, especially when a transverse Pfannenstiel incision was used. There is then a slightly more restricted access to the operation site in the uterus than there is when the abdominal incision is vertically placed.

There were various experiments with anaesthesia for caesarean section. Spinal anaesthesia was occasionally used but was condemned for the reasons mentioned above. An alternative was epidural anaesthesia with some pethidine and relaxant. The object here was mainly to allow the woman to see her baby born. Some women especially wanted to witness this, for they felt that the sight would be emotionally satisfying, at least in part like that which they hoped and expected they would feel with a vaginal delivery. There was a time when it was widely believed that fully experiencing the birth process was an essential element in the bonding which should occur between mother and baby. That is a matter difficult to prove, yet may well be valid. In any case the woman, except perhaps in emergency, should be given the opportunity to be conscious during the delivery of her baby by caesarean section.

This method of retaining consciousness was often advocated for women with cardiac disease. It avoided the need for an inhalational anaesthetic which can adversely affect some cardiac patients.

The really important trend in this period was for anaesthetists, properly trained in the needs of obstetric patients, to take over the relief of pain at all stages of labour and for operations. This was increasingly realized to be no subject for amateurs. Anaesthesia can be a major cause of death in childbirth as the national statistics showed. It was a valuable advance in care that anaesthetists were in charge of their part in the care of childbearing women in the labour wards and operating theatres. Obstetric anaesthesia as a specialty came into its own during this period, with immensely beneficial results. Of course routine sedation and analgesia could remain with midwives and obstetricians, but anything more complicated was best dealt with by those trained in the new specialty.

Puerperium

In older usage the puerperium was defined as the period during which the genital organs returned to normal after childbirth. This could take a few weeks, for after birth the uterus is a large organ weighing about 1kg, whereas in the non-pregnant woman it weighs only a few grams. To effect the changes needed for restoration to the non-pregnant state demands great metabolic activity. A silly ritual of measuring the height of the fundus of the uterus above the symphysis pubis was carried on. It was charted daily as if it gave an indication of the rate of involution. The measurement is only in one dimension whereas involution is three dimensional. It wasted a lot of time to no purpose.

The lying-in period, during which time the woman was expected to remain more or less in bed was taken to be about three weeks. In the 1950s it came to be shortened to two weeks, and later still to only a few days. The change paralleled that in surgery. Early ambulation after operations and rapid return home came to be accepted as the norm by patients and professionals. There was no doubt that men and women, over the decades, had become taller, heavier, sturdier, better educated and better housed. They were immensely healthier than their forebears. Moreover they were subjected to fewer hazards of surgery and obstetrics because of ready availability of means to combat haemorrhage and infection by transfusion, chemotherapy and antibiotics. Anaesthetics too had become less dangerous than in earlier days. The result was that after a normal birth, without complications, the woman would be up and about within hours, and ready to go home from hospital in two or three days. Even after a forceps delivery with an episiotomy she would be in hospital for no more than about five days. After a caesarean section the time of stay in hospital might be about seven days. To many older professionals these reductions in stay in hospital seemed very drastic and perhaps liable to cause problems for both mother and baby. However experience and investigation showed that problems after early discharge from hospital were very few. Most of them could be coped with at home, for midwives were required to visit daily for at least the ten days after birth. In the days following there were home calls from Health Visitors. So although professional supervision was less intensive than in hospitals it was still practised, and the monitoring of progress at home forestalled most potentially serious problems.

There were many who feared that the woman was being returned to household and family duties much too early by these newer practices. They urged that the time in hospital gave complete rest, though they ignored the fact that it was physical rest and not necessarily psychological. Most women, feeling well, wanted to get home as quickly as possible. Their wishes quite rightly prevailed. But the puerperium is by no means free of complications and problems, whether the woman is at home or in hospital or nursing home.

Infection

This is common in the genital tract, but also in the urinary tract, breasts and chest. A raised temperature may be the first indication of any of these. There could be symptoms and signs showing where the infection might be, such as abnormal lochia (the discharge from the uterus after birth), frequency and pain on micturition, engorged breasts or a cough. Signs in the chest or in the breasts were obvious enough, and there might be tenderness over the kidneys or bladder or the uterus. But although these were helpful it came to be realized that bacteriological examination was always required. This meant taking swabs from high in the vagina, and more rarely from the throat and the milk, and having a mid-stream specimen of urine examined. Also important was the examination of the calves for any signs of deep thrombosis. These investigations usually located the sites of infection which could then be treated with the appropriate antibiotic. In severe cases this was given before the microbiologist had reported on the sensitivity of any organisms grown, but in less severe cases the report could be awaited until the right antibiotic could be given. The range of these antibiotics was now so wide that infection rarely caused a great deal of anxiety in the puerperium. Yet there were a few cases where infection was fulminating and needed more drastic measures, even including surgery sometimes.

Haemorrhage

This, too, was sometimes life-threatening, though more often was just an alarming nuisance dealt with by curettage under anaesthesia, for the cause of bleeding was almost always due to a piece of retained placenta. But a few were caused by infection in a torn cervix or an episiotomy or tear. These usually required antibiotic treatment in the first instance followed perhaps by surgical repair at a later date. Blood transfusion was of course necessary in severer losses of blood.

Breastfeeding

It became recognized that the delivery of the placenta set in train several endocrine changes, as the high concentrations of oestrogens and progestogens in the blood fell rapidly. This was a stimulus for the pituitary gland to secrete prolactin for the production of milk in the breasts and for oxytocin to act on the breast causing contraction of cells round the ducts to expel the milk into the waiting mouth of the baby.

For the first few days after birth the breasts produce only colostrum, and not fully formed milk. The colostrum is valuable for the transmission of some antibodies to the baby, and the act of suckling helps to stimulate the endocrine system and is a rehearsal of breastfeeding for both mother and baby. By the fourth day after birth the milk supply often increases rapidly so that the breasts become engorged. This is a painful condition which requires relief. In the earlier days of this period the only forms of relief were by the oral administration of oestrogens, usually stilboestrol, and manual expression of the breasts to reduce the congestion. Only later was the endocrinology better understood and the preferred drug was then bromocriptine, which blocks the production and use of prolactin.

Some midwives advocated restriction of fluid intake and tight binding of the breasts for engorgement. This was naive. The intake of fluid has nothing to do with the amount secreted by the breasts, and pressure on the exterior of the breasts cannot possibly prevent the secretion pressure, which is dependent on the cells and their physiological work. However the firm support of the breasts could be comforting.

Engorgement could lead to infection, especially if the nipple was cracked as a result of the baby, or a breast pump, traumatizing it. Apart from being extremely painful such a crack opens a way into the ducts where milk is waiting as a pabulum for bacteria, which may quickly multiply. There can then be diffuse acute mastitis, sometimes mastitis more or less localized to one anatomical segment of the breast, and sometimes there may be progression to an abscess with a pocket of pus forming.

Of course everything was done to try to prevent this sequence of events. Feeding from the breast with a cracked nipple was suspended temporarily until healing had taken place. This could lead to more pain from engorgement since the milk was not being removed, except perhaps inefficiently by expression or an abhorrent nearly valueless breast pump. This was often good cause for the abandonment of breastfeeding entirely, much welcomed by the sufferer. Milk secretion was then suppressed by the use of oestrogens, which were not always very effective, but the best on offer until bromocriptine was available.

Antibiotics were of course prescribed as soon as there seemed to be evidence of infection in the breasts. It was not always easy to differentiate infection from engorgement, except by skin redness and localized tenderness. Bacteriological swabs were taken from milk expressed from the nipple. Abscesses tended to localize and showed as swelling with redness over it. The pus had to be evacuated surgically and breastfeeding abandoned.

Many women find breastfeeding abhorrent psychologically. It is important that they should not be bullied by well-meaning advisers to undertake it if they are sure of their feelings. Such women should be identified in the antenatal clinics. Some are willing to try breastfeeding but find that they too are psychologically unsuited to it. They should not be bullied either but given the quickest available route to milk suppression. Yet others passionately wish to breastfeed their babies but are unable to continue because of the pain it causes or superadded infection.

Even women who successfully breastfeed often find that the process is painful at first, perhaps for several days. It may take some fortitude to persist. If they do then they may come to enjoy breastfeeding. It gives a sense of peace and oneness with the baby. There arises a psychological bond between them which was and is thought to be valuable for the mental and emotional development of the baby. Much, perhaps too much, has been made of this concept. It does not mean that this is the only way to bonding. Bonds are established between mothers and their babies who are not breastfed. It may be easier to develop those bonds through breastfeeding, but that is not the *sine qua non* of doing so. Later in life it is not possible to differentiate the breastfed from those who were not by their psychological and emotional characteristics. There is much more to personality traits than breastfeeding and the bonding it engenders.

The majority of mothers gave up breastfeeding by about six weeks. Most of them found it more convenient to change their babies to bottle feeding with artificial milks. This was sometimes attributed to the power of advertising by the manufacturers. However it was partly a cultural phenomenon and mothers and their older relatives often persuaded each other that artificial feeds were best. They had the merit in some of their eyes that the amount of milk which the baby took was measurable. In breastfeeding this cannot be done except by test weighing which most mothers did not understand. They were not content simply to rely on the general health of the baby and steady progress in its weight gain.

On the other hand there were several women who so enjoyed breastfeeding that they found it hard to give it up. They might go on breastfeeding for up to nine months, and sometimes even longer.

The lesson for all professionals was that there was immense individal variation between women about breastfeeding. The lessons were often not heeded and there was often a near fanatical insistence by them that breastfeeding should be accomplished in all cases, whatever the odds. This zeal was taken up by journalists and authors so that those who did not breastfeed were made to feel that they had failed their babies in some way. It was unkind and unnecessary to do so, but there are always those who think they know best what is good for others and insist that their advice should be followed. There is no place for such dictatorship by professionals in the practice of midwifery. Yet that was all too often the case in the 1950s and 1960s.

There had been some rigidity in the advice given to feed the baby only every four hours. This might have seemed ideal, especially for the mother, but was rapidly abandoned by many women as soon as they could escape from the hands of the professionals. They fed their babies on demand, to the greater satisfaction of both.

Deep venous thrombosis (DVT)

After childbirth, as after surgical operations, there is a tendency for blood to clot in the deep veins of the legs and pelvis, in the latter when there is infection there. In some cases the clot is loosely attached to the vein wall and may break off to be carried in ever wider veins to the lungs as an embolus. If such an embolus is sufficiently large it may cause sudden death. Pulmonary embolism always figured as a cause of death in the national mortality statistics. It can be a major tragedy for it is so often quite unexpected in an otherwise healthy young woman.

It became routine to test all puerperal woman clinically every day for DVT. That involved deep palpation along the course of the deep veins in the calf, with the knees bent and the muscles relaxed. Tenderness suggested the possibility of DVT. Another test was to force the foot upwards with the knee extended (Homan's sign). The tightening of the muscles might cause pain in DVT, but that was found not to be as helpful as deep palpation. At first it was difficult to be sure that the diagnosis was accurate, but later there came the use of Doppler ultrasound. The probe was placed over the femoral vein and the calf was squeezed. The pulse of blood along the venous system was recorded. If there was no such pulse then the vein was presumed to be blocked by clot.

Sometimes the first evidence of a clot was the coughing and spitting up of a small amount of blood, caused by a small embolus in the lungs. This called for immediate investigation by X-ray and the exhibition of anticoagulants to prevent the clot in the legs from spreading. Clinical suspicion of thrombosis apart from the associated embolism was a reason for prescribing anticoagulants.

Infection in the pelvis could be a cause of *phlegmasia alba dolens* or painful white leg due to thrombosis especially affecting the veins of the pelvis and those of the thigh. With the early efficient treatment of infections by antibiotics it became much rarer. Infection too seemed to fix any clots to the vein walls making them less likely to break off as emboli.

Caesarean section

This form of delivery began to be the route for up to ten per cent of births. The complications are the same as for any major operation. That means lung collapse, chest infections, peritonitis, internal bleeding, wound and deep infections, and DVT. However none of these was common. The operation itself does not last long and that minimizes anaesthetic problems in the chest. The patients are healthy at the start of the operation and not suffering from any debilitating illness. It was this relative freedom from serious complications that led to the ever wider use of caesarean section to solve many obstetric problems.

The same care as after any operation was given, such as regular pulse, temperature and respiration records, together with inspection of the wound and of the lochia for abnormal discharge, and palpation of the calves for DVT. Early ambulation, often within 24 hours, was the rule to make sure that the muscle pump of the calf musculature kept blood moving along the veins, and so prevent clots forming.

Breastfeeding was begun just as in those who had had vaginal births, yet it was more difficult to establish. It was perhaps uncomfortable for the mother having the baby close to her painful abdomen, not allowing her to give full attention to the matter of feeding. But more important was that the physiological changes on which milk production depends were somehow slower to come into operation.

A point that arose after investigation was that many women who had had a caesarean section had no more babies if the one born by operation survived. It was called one child sterility. The reason was often that the husband did not wish his wife to go through the same ordeal and danger again. He had obviously had a period of great anxiety. This demonstration of yet another psychological concomitant of childbirth came as something of a surprise, though it ought not to have been, if the professionals had had more imagination and insight.

Psychology

The puerperium is a time of great mental and emotional upheaval, which demands attention, which frequently it does not get. The woman's whole life changes immeasurably. It alters her relationships with her husband especially, but also with everyone else around her. These alterations can be very upsetting and lead to depression. Indeed virtually every woman comes to suffer from what are called 'fourth day blues'. Around this time she feels miserable and weepy, largely as a result of massive changes in her hormone balances. These affect her cerebral functions and can scarcely be avoided. Her depression is made worse by well-meaning professionals and family and friends who seem unable to understand how she could be so miserable when she has just given birth to a baby to which she looked forward and was overjoyed at the time of its arrival.

It is important that she should have this phenomenon explained and discussed so that she does not sink into a continuing depression. She needs understanding and compassionate consideration. If her mood does not elevate then depression may continue for many months after the birth. This diagnosis is often missed. When made, the depression can usually be effectively treated by drugs.

At home, of course, the problems continue. The baby demands attention at all hours of day and night. The mother may be sleepless, have difficulty with breastfeeding and suffer from backache and tiredness. While breastfeeding she may suffer from abdominal pains due to the uterus contracting as a result of the oxytocin she is producing, whose main purpose is to eject milk from the breast ducts. Her perineum may be sore and cause difficulty both in micturition and defaecation. The list of her potential problems is endless.

As a result of her concentration on the baby her husband may feel alienated and fear that his wife no longer loves him. There is, naturally enough, no inclination on the part of the woman to have sexual intercourse. Just when she needs support she does not get it. It is one of life's major events and yet she is expected to carry on as if nothing very unusual has happened to her.

Postnatal

Every woman was enjoined to attend a postnatal clinic about six weeks after delivery. The intention was to be sure that all was going well. A large number of women simply did not go to these clinics. For those who did enquiry was made about their babies and their general health and the progress of breastfeeding. In the majority of cases this had already been abandoned. Physical examination included measurement of the blood pressure and the testing of the urine for sugar and protein. These were important in those who had had pre-eclampsia, renal disease or glycosuria in pregnancy, so that follow-up investigations might be set in train to see if there was continuing disease.

Abdominal examination was of value in those who had had a caesarean section to be sure that the wound was healing well. In all who had lax abdominal muscles a course of exercises, designed to help recovery of the figure, might be prescribed. Few had the time or the energy to persist with them. The same was true of physiotherapy designed to alleviate backache, which was usually accepted by women as inevitable.

Vaginal examination was directed to the healing or otherwise of any episiotomy scar or tear. The vaginal orifice might be too lax or too tight for satisfactory intercourse. Perineal exercises for the lax one could be of some help. In those where the orifice was tight they were left to discover the matter for themselves, so that revision of the repair might be carried out when they complained of dyspareunia.

Manual examination might reveal the fact that the uterus was retroverted, or somewhat larger than usual. This last was called subinvolution. It was a useless diagnosis to make for nothing could be done about it as such. One simply had to wait to see if it caused symptoms, perhaps of menorrhagia, which had to be treated in its own right later.

Much unnecessary fuss was made about retroversion too. It is present in about ten per cent of normal non-parous women. Even if acquired after childbirth it is not often a cause of symptoms. In the postnatal period it should simply be accepted, waiting to see if any symptoms do arise later. Yet there were usually unnecessary and often fruitless attempts made to put right this normal 'abnormality'. Manual corrections were made, pressing the cervix backwards and shoving up the fundus through the posterior fornix of the vagina. When this had been done a Hodge pessary was inserted, shaped so that it would maintain the uterus in the newly acquired anteverted position. When it was taken out six weeks later the uterus often flopped back into its retroverted position. More often than not it caused no problems for the woman later, and it was best left free of meddlesome interference when it caused no symptoms.

Another doubtful practice at this stage was to cauterize any cervix which showed any redness at or around the external os. This was usually called an erosion, but was more often an eversion of the lips of the cervix due to a tear in labour, and the redness was normal columnar epithelium, which was not visible in the non-parous os. Small electrically heated wires were passed to coagulate these red surfaces. It was at least painless. For some time afterwards there was some slightly purulent discharge as the cervix healed. Often on return to the clinic the red area was seen to be covered with squamous epithelium. The obstetrician was usually satisfied by this but the woman noticed no difference. In most instances the intervention was unnecessary, and the lesion remained unhealed with this minor intervention.

It was, of course, quite different if the woman complained of a muco-purulent discharge from the cervix which was inconveniencing her. This came from the exposed columnar epithelium. It was then helpful to cauterize the cervix under anaesthesia. At a later period these lesions could be effectively treated with cold cryocautery, administered in out-patients without the need for anaesthesia.

The best reason for any postnatal consultations was the opportunity to discuss contraception and its methods. However this was just as well done by trained general practitioners and the numerous birth control clinics which had sprung up. It did not require a hospital visit.

There are trends in the 1990s to discard routine postnatal clinics. They should be selective for a few patients to review any diseases which had complicated the pregnancy and to discuss the obstetric future with those women who had had operative deliveries or who had suffered a stillbirth or neonatal death. Such women need continuing care of which the postnatal visit is only the beginning. Most of the earlier investigations and treatments were superfluous.

Health of the fetus

Through the ages there has always been concern for the welfare of the fetus and newborn. That, after all, is the proximate purpose of reproduction. It was hoped that by looking after the mother the baby would be cared for too. Indeed there was little else to be done. The embryo and fetus are locked away out of sight in a closed world that for several centuries it seemed impossible to explore and penetrate.

It is only in the 20th century that it has been possible to look more closely into the physiology and pathology of the intrauterine environment and to understand rather more precisely what goes on there.

Embryology has been a sphere of study for anatomists and biologists for a long time. It established the patterns of human and animal development in the early weeks after fertilization. How that happened was not really known until 1827 when Carl Ernst von Baer (1792–1876) first saw the ovum of a bitch. He also described the three germ layers of the early embryo more exactly than before. The place of genetics in development began to be understood by Gregor Mendel (1822–1884), the monk of Brno (now Brünn) in Czechoslovakia, with his famous experiments on the inheritance of greenness, yellowness, smoothness and wrinkliness in peas. Despite his work in the 1850s it did not come to general scientific notice until 1900.

Wilhelm Roux (1850–1924) of Halle described the chromosomes of the nucleus of cells as the instruments of heredity in 1883. Later there followed the descriptions of cell division as meiosis in the production of the germ cells, and of mitosis in all other cellular replications. The intermediate processes as to how the genes on the chromosomes controlled development had to wait for James Dewey Watson (b.1928) and Francis Harry Compton Crick (b.1916) along with several others who determined the nature and structure of DNA (desoxyribose nucleic acid) in 1953. That seminal work, now part of the folklore of science, in turn depended on previous investigations in biochemistry, X-ray crystallography and physics showing the importance of spatial arrangements of atoms within molecules and how they could all react with one another.

Clinically it was well-known that certain diseases and deformities were inherited, but exactly how those came about was not known, though it is being intensively investigated in the last quarter of the 20th century. Genes causing many diseases have been located precisely in a variety of chromosomes, and there is a worldwide drive to map the whole of the human genome, so that each gene locus may be identified as being responsible for some or other characteristic of the individual as an infant, child and adult.

In the period just after 1950 it was thought that there was no way to offset genetic diseases. They were deemed to be inbuilt, and so incapable of being influenced. Then came the remarkable clinical work (1941) of Norman McAlister Gregg (1892–1966) of Sydney, an ophthalmologist, who noted that a cluster of congenital cataracts in children coincided with their mothers suffering from rubella (German measles) in early pregnancy. Such infection can cause blindness, deafness and cardiac anomalies in the newborn and child. Thus infection could interfere with development by altering the genes in some way. Then came the discovery that the drug thalidomide, administered in early pregnancy for sickness, could cause failure of development of some or all of the limbs. Many other drugs and infections, such as measles, mumps, toxoplasmosis, cytomegalovirus, came under suspicion of being similarly damaging. Since so little was then known about any of them, it became important to shield pregnant women from contact with viral diseases especially, and from the administration of drugs except those strictly necessary for the treatment of diseases in the mother. Even among these there were dangers, for phenylhydantoin, widely used for the control of epilepsy was shown to have teratogenic effects. Various treatments of thyroid disorder have effects on the fetus too.

So damaging was rubella to the baby that pregnant women were advised to avoid contact with children at risk, though this was not always possible when there were other children in the family. Then there was routine investigation of rubella antibodies for all women to determine if they had had silent or undiagnosed infection with the disease earlier. Those who did not have antibodies were given rubella vaccine to stimulate production of them so that they would protect against the infection. Such vaccination was then extended to cover all girls aged about 11 or 12 so that their later offspring would be protected from infection in pregnancy.

Another earlier routine investigation in pregnancy was that of testing the mother's blood for previous syphilis by the Wassermann reaction or later modifications of that test. It was important to treat any syphilis early in pregnancy in order to protect the fetus. Syphilitic mothers tended to have a series of stillbirths, and any liveborn babies were sickly and had the stigmata of the congenital disease in a saddle nose, with 'snuffles', notched teeth, skin eruptions, pseudoparalysis due to bone disease and many other unpleasant clinical manifestations. In the 1990s syphilis in pregnancy is rare because of the relatively easy and efficacious treatment of the disease in non-pregnant women by penicillin and other drugs. From these examples it can be seen that the health of fetuses can be partly assured from treatments and specific diagnoses made before pregnancy.

After the early differentiation of organs and tissues in the embryo the later stages of pregnancy are essentially concerned with growth. Fetuses that have a birthweight in the region of 7lbs or 3.4kg are known to have the best chances of survival to a later age. By measuring the weights of babies born at various times of gestation, growth curves were established together with their normal deviations. The problem, of course, after this was to determine the weight of the fetus in utero. For a long time this estimate had to be made by clinical guesswork, based to some extent on experience. But it was notoriously inaccurate.

Fetal growth depends on the integrity of the placenta, so that there came the concept of the feto-placental unit. In cases of clinical doubt about the welfare of the fetus and just how well it was growing placental function was investigated by hormone assays on maternal urine and blood. Later came sonar (ultrasound) which could directly measure some parts of the fetus. These have been discussed earlier.

Apart from the actual cellular structure of the placenta its function depends on both the maternal blood flow and fetal blood flow to it. These are almost impossible at present to measure clinically. Much physiological work however has been done on animals concerning these parameters. They have helped to illuminate some clinical thinking about pregnancy problems. Other physiological animal experiments have given indications of how various nutrients, excretory products and the respiratory gases of oxygen and carbon dioxide cross to each side of the placenta. Again such investigations are not possible in pregnancy, though samples of maternal and of fetal blood taken at caesarean section have helped to verify the general applicability of the animal work to the human.

With an otherwise normal fetus its growth depends essentially on the maternal blood supply to the placenta. Little is directly known about this, but since fetal growth is slowed in certain conditions of the mother, such as essential hypertension and pre-eclampsia it is assumed that these are associated with reduced maternal blood flow. Better pharmacological agents than we have now should be able to improve the blood flow and so perhaps aid fetal growth.

The general nutritional state of the mother has some influence on the weight of the baby at birth, though less than might at first be imagined. Tall and heavy women tend to have statistically larger babies, while short and slim women have smaller ones. However in advanced societies extra supplements of nutrients for mothers may have little effect. Many of these have been tried, such as milk and vitamins but they do not always seem to be successful in preventing the birth of small babies. Even gross starvation which was seen in some Nazi concentration camps did not seriously lower the birth weights of babies until the mothers weighed about 7 stone (44.5kg) or under. The fetus therefore seems able to extract what it needs from the mother's blood even at her expense.

In animals there is some evidence that lack of certain specific elements in the food, such as riboflavin, at certain crucial points in pregnancy may result in embryonic and fetal abnormalities, but the evidence for such effects is not so certain for humans.

The actual size of the placenta and the number of cells it contains could obviously be a limiting factor on growth. In normal pregnancy there is a rough 7:1 ratio between the weights of the baby and the placenta. Presumably a small placenta could only support the growth of a small baby. But the determinants of the size and weight of the placenta are not known. Intensive pathological and histological investigation of the placenta after delivery shows some changes in hypertension and pre-eclampsia. There are small parts of the placenta where the blood supply from the maternal side has been cut off and caused death of the cells in those areas. But these anatomical changes only rarely seem to be enough to be a cause of impaired growth of the fetus, unless they are massive. They are probably only an indication of generalized poor blood supply, worse in these obviously affected areas.

A big problem for understanding the nature of the work of the placenta is that under the microscope it is essentially a simple structure. There are two layers of cells, one with cell boundaries and the other without them. They are very large sheets in total area because they are thrown up into arborising processes called villi, which dip like the roots of trees into the maternal blood lake. How this apparently simple structure can carry out the multiple functions that it does is by no means fully known yet. It is a major key to the understanding of the nature of the intrauterine life and health of the fetus.

There can be no doubt that poor placental function can result in the death of the fetus. It is obvious in the acute separation of the placenta in abruptio placentae. More chronically death can occur by slow starvation as the placenta fails to meet the needs of the growing fetus. This is the cause of the small-for-dates baby. It is important to recognize it in pregnancy for the sooner the fetus is out of its deteriorating environment, whatever the cause, the better. There is a greater chance of the baby's survival in the Special Care Baby Unit than in the womb.

There are cases where the baby may grow almost too large. This may happen if pregnancy is unduly prolonged perhaps to 42 or more weeks. If too large they too may run out of adequate nutritional support despite their size, because of relative placental failure in supplying their needs. They too may require delivery as soon as the potential problem is recognized. A well-known cause of big babies is maternal diabetes. If this is not controlled there is a tendency for the babies to be overweight for the length of gestation. Many of them are stillborn and the incidence of abnormalities is higher than average. They tend to be sickly at birth and need special medical and nursing attention. This is a good example of the need to keep the mother as healthy as possible so that the intrauterine environment may be as optimal as can be.

The embryo and fetus need protection from being expelled early from the uterus, before they have had time to come to maturity and so may have difficulty in surviving in the outside world. The causes of early expulsion are largely unknown. Abortion or miscarriage in the early weeks affects up to about ten per cent of all pregnancies. It is thought, by examination after expulsion, that many of them are due to embryonic abnormalities of genetic origin, and others due to some hormone imbalance. There seems no way to prevent the genetic causes. Several attempts have been made to correct supposed failure in the production of progesterone as a cause of abortion, but this has not met with universal success.

At a later stage in pregnancy there is a tendency to lose the baby if the cervix has been severely torn in a previous pregnancy or after a too vigorous dilatation operatively. A stitch passed round the lax part of the internal os of the cervix (Shirodkar) usually prevents early expulsion in the mid-trimester. The stitch is removed when maturity has been reached or if the woman goes into labour.

Premature labour, prior to the beginning of the 38th week of pregnancy is not fully understood. Nor is the onset of labour at term. It may be controlled by endocrine secretions from the fetal glands, perhaps its adrenals. These might then stimulate the posterior lobe of the pituitary of the mother to secrete oxytocin, which causes uterine contractions. Sometimes rest alone may prevent the progress of such early labours, and drugs such as salbutamol and alcohol have had some limited success. Provided however that the baby weighs about 5lbs (2.5kg) or more it nowadays has good chances of survival, since the paediatric care of the newborn has so massively improved over the last few decades. There is therefore less need than there used to be to try to prevent progress in labour, provided that pregnancy has lasted about 34–35 weeks.

A major advance has been in the recognition of various forms of Rhesus incompatibility between the fetus and the mother. The outline of this disorder has been described earlier. In some cases where the fetal blood group is Rhesus positive and the mother's is Rhesus negative she reacts to her fetus by producing Rhesus antibodies. These cross the placenta and slowly destroy the fetal cells by haemolysis. The result is that the fetus becomes progressively anaemic. This may be so severe as to cause cardiac failure and the baby may die showing massive oedema – *hydrops fetalis*. In babies born alive they too may be anaemic and rapidly develop jaundice which can threaten some brain cells and cause mental retardation.

The brilliant work of Professor Sir Cyril Clarke of Liverpool along with others has now provided the means of prevention of *erythroblastosis fetalis*, which is the name that covers all these haemolytic manifestations. Fetal red cells cross over into the mother's bloodstream mainly as the placenta is born or at the time of an abortion. Such cells which would cause the production of Rhesus antibodies can be destroyed by the injection of antibodies almost immediately after the chorionic or placental tissue is delivered. This kills off the Rhesus positive cells which have gained access to the mother before they have a chance to excite her immune system to produce antibodies. Such injections are now given to every Rhesus negative woman after an abortion or birth and the result has been virtually to banish erythroblastosis in the fetus. This is a remarkable example of preventive medicine. It protects further fetuses from damage in subsequent pregnancies.

Many genetic diseases tend to manifest themselves after birth when they are based on enzyme disorders such as those of adrenal hyperplasia. Some of these disorders tend to recur in second and later pregnancies. If so these babies can be recognized in utero before they are born. This is done by withdrawing liquor amnii with a needle through the abdominal wall for biochemical analysis. Paediatric physicians can then be alerted to the problem and be ready to deal with it immediately after birth. Paediatricians and geneticists increasingly guide obstetricians in the management of pregnancy in the interests of the fetus and newborn.

Some serious congenital defects in the fetus can be picked up by ultrasound investigations quite early in pregnancy. Although counsel of despair the parents can then be offered a termination of pregnancy. The decision to do this is much more difficult to make in later pregnancy when excessive amounts of liquor amnii (hydramnios) may indicate that the fetus is abnormal. X-rays may confirm it.

Also difficult in deciding what to do is when fetal cells taken by amniocentesis of the liquor indicate the possibility of the trisomy of Down's syndrome. Such tests are often performed on older mothers where the risk is higher. Children with this disorder are born alive yet are mentally retarded. They may live for several decades. It is an agonising decision as to whether the pregnancy should be terminated or allowed to continue, knowing the burden the abnormality will certainly impose on parents.

One of the major causes of death in the neonatal period is respiratory distress syndrome, which especially affects premature babies. It is associated with abnormalities in the lecithin:sphingomyelin ratio in the liquor amnii. The changes can be reversed by the administration of corticosteroids to the mother prior to the birth. In premature labours liquor is withdrawn and analysed for these two substances so that appropriate treatment may be given to prevent the respiratory distress syndrome.

Obviously the care of the fetus is especially intensified during labour. It is a time when acute anoxia can occur, causing fetal distress, which may demand immediate delivery. Such is especially needed when the umbilical cord prolapses, causing arrest of the fetal circulation. There are less acute causes of anoxia due to vigorous uterine contractions which can seriously diminish the flow through the maternal side of the placenta. Or premature separation of the placenta may have the same effect.

Fetal anoxia is clinically recognized by changes in the fetal heart rate which is routinely recorded clinically in labour. It has already been mentioned that more precise logging of the rate may be made by fetal electrocardiography. That may be supplemented by sampling of the fetal blood taken from the scalp when the cervix is open so that its oxygen content and its hydrogen ion content can be determined.

It has been emphasized how attention in obstetrics has gradually moved over the years from being concerned almost entirely with the mother's health so that it now includes that of her fetus just as much, and has done for some decades. It is not that the fetus was ignored in previous history, but rather that there was little that could be done for it when things went wrong. Moreover there was the attitude that the fetus was expendable if the mother's survival depended on it. While making efforts to save the baby this was of secondary importance to that of the mother. If she lived she could reproduce again, perhaps more successfully. If she died that particular family ceased. That has now changed. There are few situations where the obstetric interests of the mother seriously conflict with those of her fetus nowadays. Both are of much more equal concern than they ever were in bygone days.

Of course birth is only one major incident in any life history. There is an unbroken progress from fertilization to death, at whatever age that may occur. There is medical specialization at every stage in life. The complete generalist in medicine was probably always a myth. Now it is certainly seen to be. Whereas the obstetrician, even in the 1950s, was often the person looking after the newborn, that is no longer the case. The paediatricians take over from the moment of birth. They have developed methods and techniques of immense erudition. The development and history of these is beyond the purview of this book. But paediatricians have contributed to obstetric practice in that their expertise has made it possible to end difficult and doubtful cases of pregnancy much before the time that was once possible. Babies used to be in danger if delivered before about the 37th week of pregnancy. Now they more often than not survive even if they are born as early as the 34th week and often much earlier than this.

Bibliography

Bynum, W.F. and Porter, R. (Eds). (1985). *William Hunter and the Eighteenth Century Medical World*. Cambridge: Cambridge University Press.

Castiglioni, A. (1947). *A History of Medicine*. 2nd edn. London: Routledge and Kegan Paul.

Catalogue and Report of Obstetrical and other Instruments. (1867). London: Longmans, Green and Co.

Chapman, E. (1735). *A Treatise on the Improvement of Midwifery*. London: John Brindley.

Crainz, F. (1977). *An Obstetric Tragedy*. London: Heinemann Medical Books Ltd.

Cullingworth, C.J. (1904). *Charles White, F.R.S.* London: Henry J. Glaisher.

Cunningham, A. and French, R. (Eds). (1990). *The Medical Enlightenment of the Eighteenth Century*. Cambridge: Cambridge University Press.

Dewhurst, J. (1980). *Royal Confinements*. London: Weidenfeld & Nicolson.

Eccles, A. (1982). *Obstetrics and Gynaecology in Tudor and Stuart England*. London: Croom Helm.

Fairley, P. (1982). *The Conquest of Pain*. 2nd impression. London: Michael Joseph.

Fisher, R.B. (1977). *Joseph Lister 1827–1912*. London: Macdonald and Jane's.

Fleetwood Churchill (Ed). (1849). *Essays on the Puerperal Fever*. London: Sydenham Society.

French, R. and Wear, A. (Eds). (1989). *The Medical Revolution of the Seventeenth Century*. Cambridge: Cambridge University Press.

Garrison, F.H. (1929). *An Introduction to the History of Medicine*. 4th edn. Philadelphia: W.B. Saunders & Co.

Graham, H. (1950). *Eternal Eve*. London: Heinemann Medical Books.

Greenhill, J.P., Pitkin, R.M. and Zlatnik, F.J. (1955–1981). Obstetrics and Gynecology Year Books. Chicago: Year Book Medical Publishers Inc.

Guthrie, D. (1945). *A History of Medicine*. Walton on Thames: Thomas Nelson and Sons Ltd.

Hagelin, O. (1990). *The Byrth of Mankynde otherwise named The Woman's Booke*. An illustrated and annotated Catalogue of rare books in the library of the Swedish Society of Medicine, Stockholm.

Haggard, H.W. (No date). *Devils, Drugs and Doctors*. London: Heinemann Medical Books Ltd.

HMSO (1952–54, 1955–57, 1958–60, 1961–63, 1964–66, 1967–69, 1970–72, 1973–75). *Confidential Enquiries into Maternal Deaths in England and Wales*. London: HMSO.

Holy Bible. (1974). New International Version. New York International Bible Society. London: Hodder and Stoughton.

Illingworth, C. (1967). *The Story of William Hunter*. Edinburgh: E. & S. Livingstone Ltd.

Johnstone, R.W. (1952). *William Smellie*. Edinburgh: E. & S. Livingstone Ltd.

Keynes, G. (1949). *The Personality of William Harvey*. Cambridge: Cambridge University Press.

Lloyd, G.E.R. (Ed). (1978). *The Hippocratic Writings*. London: Pelican Books.

Mill, J.S. (1955). *The Subjection of Women*. London: J.M. Dent & Sons Ltd.

Morton, H.V. (1956). *Women of the Bible*. London. Methuen & Co. Ltd.

Morton, L.T. (1983). *A Medical Bibliography*. 4th edn. Aldershot: Gower Publishing Company.

Moscucci, O. (1990). *The Science of Woman 1800–1929*. Cambridge: Cambridge University Press.

Munro Kerr, J.M., Johnstone, R.W. and Phillips, M.H. (Eds). (1954). *Historical Review of British Obstetrics and Gynaecology 1800–1950*. Edinburgh: E. & S. Livingstone Ltd.

Newman, C. (1957). *The Evolution of Medical Education in the Nineteenth Century*. Oxford: Oxford University Press.

Obstetric Plates (1837). Selected from *The Anatomical Tables of William Smellie*. London: Samuel Highley.

Parry-Jones, E. (1972). *Barton's Forceps.* London: Sector Publishing Ltd.

Peterson, M.J. (1978). *The Medical Profession in Mid-Victorian London.* California: University of California Press.

Poidevin, L.O.S. (1965). *Caesarean Section Scars.* Springfield, Ill.: Chas. C. Thomas.

Porter, I.A. (1958). *Alexander Gordon. M.D. of Aberdeen 1752-1799.* Edinburgh: Oliver and Boyd.

Radcliffe, W. (1947). *The Secret Instrument.* London: Heinemann Medical Books Ltd.

Reiser, S.J. (1978). *Medicine and the Reign of Technology.* Cambridge: Cambridge University Press.

Rhodes, P. (1977). *Dr John Leake's Hospital.* London: Davis-Poynter.

Rhodes, P. (1985). *An Outline History of Medicine.* London: Butterworth.

Rivett, G. (1986). *The Development of the London Hospital System 1823-1982.* London: King Edward' Hospital Fund for London.

Roodhouse Gloyne, S. (1950). *John Hunter.* Edinburgh: E. & S. Livingstone.

Rossetti, L. (1983). *The University of Padua.* Trieste: Edizioni Lint.

Seltman, C. (1956). *Women in Antiquity.* London: Pan Books Ltd.

Shepherd, J.A. (1965). *Spencer Wells.* Edinburgh: E. & S. Livingstone.

Shryock, R.H. (1974). *The Development of Modern Medicine.* Wisconsin, USA: The University of Wisconsin Press.

Simpson, M. (1972). *Simpson the Obstetrician.* London: Victor Gollancz.

Singer, C. (1928). *A Short History of Medicine.* Oxford: Oxford at the Clarendon Press.

Singer, C. and Underwood, E. A. (1962). *A Short History of Medicine.* Oxford: Oxford at the Clarendon Press.

Smellie, W. (1974). *A Treatise on the Theory and Practice of Midwifery. 1752.* Facsimile edn. London: Scolar Press.

Speert, H. (1958). *Obstetric and Gynecologic Milestones.* New York: The Macmillan Company.

Speert, H. (1973). *Iconographia Gyniatrica.* Philadelphia, USA: F.A. Davis Company.

Spencer, H.R. (1927). *The History of British Midwifery from 1650 to 1800.* London: John Bale, Sons & Danielsson Ltd.

Spratt, G. (1833). *Obstetric Tables.* London. John Churchill.

Stroganoff, W. (1930). *The Improved Prophylactic Method in the Treatment of Eclampsia.* Edinburgh: E. & S. Livingstone Ltd.

Thoms, H. (1935). *Classical Contributions to Obstetrics and Gynecology.* Springfield, Ill.: Chas. C. Thomas.

Waddington, I. (1984). *The Medical Profession in the Industrial Revolution.* Dublin: Gill and Macmillan Ltd.

Walton, J., Beeson, P.B. and Bodley Scott, R. (1986). *The Oxford Companion to Medicine.* Vols. I and II. Oxford: Oxford University Press.

Webster, C. (1979). *Health, Medicine and Mortality in the Sixteenth Century.* Cambridge: Cambridge University Press.

Willey, B. (1962). *The Seventeenth Century Background.* London: Peregrine (Penguin Books).

Willey, B. (1964). *The Eighteenth Century Background.* London: Penguin Books.

Willughby, P. (1972). *Observations in Midwifery.* Wakefield: S.R. Publishers Ltd.

Wollstonecraft, M. (1955). *The Rights of Woman.* London: J.M. Dent & Sons Ltd.

Zinsser, H. (1937). *Rats, Lice and History.* London: Routledge & Sons. Ltd.

Index

M